MICROWAVE RECIPES 2022

DELICIOUS AND HEALTHY RECIPES FOR BUSY PEOPLE

JOHN ASHES

Table of Contents

Chocolate Fondue

Serves 3–4

200 g/7 oz plain (semi-sweet) chocolate

150 ml/¼ pt/2/3 cup double (heavy) cream

15 ml/1 tbsp whisky, rum, brandy or orange-flavoured liqueur or 5 ml/1 tsp vanilla essence (extract)

Small biscuits, marshmallows and/or pieces of fresh fruit, to serve

Break up the chocolate and place in a basin. Melt, uncovered, on Defrost for 4–5 minutes until soft. Stir in the cream and heat, uncovered, on Defrost for about 1½ minutes. Stir in the alcohol or vanilla essence. Serve warm with biscuits, marshmallows and/or fresh fruit pieces for dipping.

Orange Chocolate Fondue

Serves 3–4

Prepare as for Chocolate Fondue, but use only Grand Marnier, Mandarine Napolean liqueur or Cointreau. Flavour with 5 ml/1 tsp finely grated orange peel.

Mocha Fondue

Serves 3–4

Prepare as for Chocolate Fondue, but add 15 ml/1 tbsp instant coffee powder with the cream and use only Tia Maria, Kahlua or coffee essence (extract) to flavour.

White Chocolate Fondue

Serves 3–4

Prepare as for Chocolate Fondue, but substitute white chocolate for the plain (semi-sweet) and add 30 ml/2 tbsp of the measured cream to the chocolate before melting. Flavour with vanilla essence (extract) or an orange liqueur instead of the suggested spirits.

Toblerone Fondue

Serves 3–4

Prepare as for Chocolate Fondue, but substitute white, milk or dark Toblerone chocolate for the plain (semi-sweet) chocolate.

Royal Chocolate Mousse

Makes 10–12

15 ml/1 tbsp powdered gelatine

150 ml/¼ pt/2/3 cup cold water

500 g/1 lb 2 oz plain (semi-sweet) chocolate (70% cocoa)

30 ml/2 tbsp butter

75 ml/3 fl oz/5½ tbsp strong hot coffee

4 eggs, at kitchen temperature, separated

A pinch of salt

Coffee or cocoa (unsweetened chocolate) powder, to serve

Soak the gelatine in a glass jug in cold water 5 minutes. Melt, uncovered, on Full for 1½–2 minutes until the liquid looks clear. Stir round, then set aside. Break up the chocolate and place in a fairly large bowl with the butter and coffee. Melt, uncovered, on Defrost for 6–7 minutes. Stir in the egg yolks and melted gelatine. Chill until just beginning to thicken and set slightly round the edges. Whisk together the egg whites and salt until they form stiff peaks. Beat one-third into the chocolate mixture, then gently and smoothly fold in the remainder. Divide between 10–12 ramekin dishes (custard cups). Chill for several hours until firm. Dust with coffee or cocoa powder before serving.

Dutch-style Pears with Chocolate Advocaat Mousse

Serves 6

10 ml/2 tsp powdered gelatine

30 ml/2 tbsp cold water

100 g/3½ oz plain (semi-sweet) chocolate

2 eggs, at kitchen temperature, separated

150 ml/¼ pt/2/3 cup advocaat (egg liqueur)

425 g/15 oz/1 large can pear halves in juice or syrup, drained

30 ml/2 tbsp chopped pistachio nuts

Soak the gelatine in a glass jug in cold water for 5 minutes. Melt, uncovered, on Full for 1–1½ minutes until the liquid looks clear. Stir round and set aside. Break up the chocolate and place in a separate bowl. Melt, uncovered, on Defrost for 3–3½ minutes. Stir well. Mix in the dissolved gelatine, egg yolks and advocaat. Beat until smooth and evenly combined. Cover and chill until just beginning to thicken and set. Beat the egg whites to stiff peaks. Whisk one-third into the chocolate mixture, then fold in the remainder with a metal spoon. Divide the pears between six sundae glasses and top evenly with the chocolate mixture. Chill until set. Sprinkle with the nuts before serving.

Traditional Chocolate Mousse

Serves 4

100 g/3½ oz plain (semi-sweet) chocolate

15 ml/1 tbsp unsalted (sweet) butter

4 eggs at kitchen temperature, separated

A pinch of salt

Sponge finger biscuits (cookies), to serve

Break up chocolate, then put in a 1.25 litre/2¼ pt/5½ cup basin with the butter. Heat, uncovered, on Defrost for 3½–4 minutes, stirring once or twice, until both have melted. Mix in the egg yolks. In a separate bowl, beat the egg whites and salt to stiff peaks. Beat one-third into the chocolate mixture, then smoothly stir in the remainder with a large metal spoon. Spoon into four stemmed wine glasses. Cover with kitchen paper and chill thoroughly. Eat with sponge fingers.

Chocolate Orange Mousse

Serves 4

Prepare as for Traditional Chocolate Mousse, but add 10 ml/2 tsp finely grated orange peel with the egg yolks.

Mocha Mousse

Serves 4

Prepare as for Traditional Chocolate Mousse, but add 10 ml/2 tsp instant coffee granules with the egg yolks.

Chocolate Peppermint Cream Mousse

Serves 4

Prepare as for Traditional Chocolate Mousse, but add a few drops of peppermint essence (extract) with the egg yolks. Just before serving, decorate the top of each with whipped cream.

Berlin Air

Serves 6–8

Germany's answer to Italy's zabaglione and Britain's syllabub.

4 large eggs, separated
A pinch of salt
150 g/5 oz/2/3 cup caster (superfine) sugar
5 ml/1 tsp vanilla essence (extract)
10 ml/2 tsp cornflour (cornstarch)
150 ml/¼ pt/2/3 cup sweet white wine
150 ml/¼ pt/2/3 cup double (heavy) cream
30 ml/2 tbsp brandy
Wafer biscuits (cookies) and mixed berry fruits (optional), to serve

Whisk the egg whites with the salt until stiff. Whisk together the yolks, sugar and vanilla in a large bowl until the mixture is pale and thick. Gently whisk in the whites. Mix the cornflour smoothly with a little of the wine, then stir in the remainder. Fold into the egg mixture. Cook, uncovered, on Full for 3½ minutes, whisking every 30 seconds, until the mixture is foaming and resembles thickish custard. Cover and leave until completely cold. In large bowl, whisk the cream with the brandy until thick. Gradually whisk in the egg mixture. Spoon into six to eight individual ramekin dishes (custard cups) and chill thoroughly. Serve with crisp wafer biscuits and accompany, in season, with fresh berry fruits.

Crème Caramel

Serves 4

Prepare one quantity of Baked Egg Custard. Pour bought caramel sauce into four buttered ramekin dishes (custard cups) and top with the egg custard. Cook, uncovered, on Defrost for 8–9 minutes until the custard is set. Allow to cool, then chill thoroughly. Turn out on to individual plates and serve with cream.

Spicy Peaches and Oranges in Red Wine

Serves 6–8

8 large ripe peaches, blanched and skinned

Lemon juice

300 ml/½ pt/1¼ cups dry red wine

175 g/6 oz/¾ cup caster (superfine) sugar

5 cm/2 in piece cinnamon stick

4 whole cloves

2 cardamom pods

2 oranges, unpeeled and thinly sliced

Halve the peaches and twist to separate. Remove the stones (pits). Brush the flesh all over with lemon juice. Put the remaining ingredients except the oranges in a deep 20 cm/8 in diameter dish. Cover with an inverted plate and heat on Full for 4 minutes. Stir to mix. Add the peaches, cut sides down, and arrange the orange slices randomly between. Cover with clingfilm (plastic wrap) and slit it twice to allow steam to escape. Cook on Full for 10 minutes, turning the dish twice. Cool and chill before serving.

Spicy Pears and Oranges in Red Wine

Serves 6–8

Prepare as for Spicy Peaches and Oranges in Red Wine, but substitute 8 small dessert pears, peeled, halved and cored, for the peaches.

Store-cupboard Raspberry Mousse

Serves 6

15 ml/1 tbsp powdered gelatine

30 ml/2 tbsp cold water

425 g/15 oz/1 large can raspberries in syrup, drained and syrup reserved

3 eggs, separated

45 ml/3 tbsp caster (superfine) sugar

A pinch of salt

150 ml/¼ pt/2/3 cup whipping cream

15 ml/1 tbsp toasted and chopped hazelnuts, to decorate

Put the gelatine in a jug with the cold water. Stir round and leave for 5 minutes to soften. Melt, uncovered, on Full for 2 minutes until the liquid is clear. Add the raspberry syrup to the gelatine. Gently beat in the egg yolks and sugar. Cover and chill until just beginning to thicken and set. Beat the egg whites and salt until stiff. Whip the cream until thick. Beat one-third of the egg whites into the gelatine mixture, then mix in two-thirds of the raspberries and three-quarters of the cream. Fold in the remaining whites with a metal spoon. When smooth and well-combined, transfer to six dessert dishes. Cover and chill until set. Before serving, stir the remaining cream into the remaining raspberries and use to decorate the top of the mousses.

Egg Custard, Apricot and Sherry Trifle

Serves 8

600 ml/1 pt/2½ cups full-cream milk or half single (light) cream and half milk

15 ml/1 tbsp cornflour (cornstarch)

15 ml/1 tbsp cold water

4 large eggs

75 ml/5 tbsp caster (superfine) sugar

5 ml/1 tsp vanilla essence (extract)

2 jam (conserve)-filled Swiss (jelly) rolls, thinly sliced

425 g/15 oz/1 large can apricot halves, drained

30 ml/2 tbsp sweet sherry

60 ml/4 tbsp apricot syrup

150 ml/¼ pt/2/3 cup double (heavy) cream

Hundreds and thousands, to decorate

Pour the milk into a jug. Warm, uncovered, on Full for 2 minutes. Put the cornflour and water in a 1.25 litre/2¼ pt/5½ cup bowl and stir until smooth. Beat in the eggs one at a time. Add 45 ml/3 tbsp of the caster sugar and mix in the warm milk. Cook, uncovered, on Full for 5–6 minutes, whisking every minute, until the custard is of a thin coating consistency (it thickens on cooling). Mix in the vanilla. Cover and set aside. Stand eight slices of Swiss roll against the side of a deep 20 cm/8 in diameter glass serving dish. Reserve 8 apricot halves for decoration and coarsely chop the remainder. Use to cover the base of the dish with the remaining Swiss roll. Moisten with the sherry and apricot syrup. Coat with half the warm custard and let it soak well in. Pour the remaining custard over the top. Cover and chill for 4–5 hours. Before serving, beat together the cream and remaining caster sugar until thick. Use to decorate the top of the trifle, then arrange the reserved apricot halves on top. Dust with hundreds and thousands.

Short-cut Sherry Trifle

Serves 6–8

1 jam (conserve)-filled Swiss (jelly) roll, thinly sliced

45 ml/3 tbsp sweet sherry

425 g/15 oz/1 large can peach slices or fruit cocktail, drained and syrup reserved

45 ml/3 tbsp custard powder

30 ml/2 tbsp caster (superfine) sugar

600 ml/1 pt/2½ cups cold milk

150 ml/¼ pt/2/3 cup whipped cream

Hundreds and thousands and red glacé (candied) cherries

Arrange the Swiss roll slices over the base and half-way up the side of a shallow glass bowl. Moisten with the sherry and few spoonfuls of the reserved syrup. Cover with the drained fruit. Put the custard powder and sugar in a fairly deep dish and mix smoothly with a little of the cold milk. Blend in the remainder. Cook, uncovered, on Full for 8 minutes, whisking briskly every minute to keep the custard smooth. Allow to cool slightly, then pour over the trifle. Cover when cold and chill thoroughly. Before serving, decorate with the whipped cream, hundreds and thousands and glacé cherries.

Note: use up any left-over syrup in fresh fruit salad.

Chocolate Cream Trifle

Serves 8

Prepare as for Egg Custard, Apricot and Sherry Trifle, but use 2 cream-filled chocolate Swiss (jelly) rolls instead of jam-filled. Substitute coffee liqueur for the sherry and canned pear halves for the apricots. Sprinkle with grated chocolate or a crushed flake bar instead of the hundreds and thousands.

Trifle with Sponge Cakes

Serves 6–8

Make any of the three trifles above, but substitute bought sponge cakes (8 in a packet) for the Swiss (jelly) roll. Split and fill with jam (conserve), curd or chocolate spread.

Fluffy Lemon Clouds

Serves 4–5

300 ml/½ pt/1¼ cups cold milk

25 ml/1½ tbsp custard powder

15 ml/1 tbsp caster (superfine) sugar

2 large eggs, separated

1 packet lemon jelly (jello)

A pinch of salt

Seasonal fruits, to decorate

Blend some of the cold milk smoothly with the custard powder in a large bowl. Mix in the remainder. Cook, uncovered, on Full for 3–3½ minutes, whisking every minute to prevent lumps forming, until the mixture comes to the boil and thickens. Beat in the sugar and egg yolks. Cover with a piece of clingfilm (plastic wrap), placing it directly on the surface of the custard to stop a skin forming. Allow to cool. Break up the jelly into cubes. Put in a measuring jug with 60 ml/4 tbsp water. Cover with a saucer and melt on Defrost for 2–2½ minutes, stirring twice. Make up to 300 ml/½ pt/1¼ cups with cold water. Lift the clingfilm off the custard and beat in the melted jelly. Cover and chill until the mixture is beginning to thicken and set. Whisk the egg whites and salt until stiff. Beat one-third into the jelly mixture, then smoothly fold in the remainder with a large metal spoon or balloon whisk. Transfer to four or five dessert glasses or dishes. Cover and chill until firm and set. Decorate with fresh seasonal fruits.

Fluffy Lime Clouds

Serves 4–5

Prepare as for Fluffy Lemon Clouds, but substitute lime jelly (jello) for the lemon.

Apple Snow

Serves 4

30 ml/2 tbsp vanilla-flavoured blancmange powder
450 ml/¾ pt/2 cups cold milk
45 ml/3 tbsp caster (superfine) sugar
125 g/4 oz/½ cup smooth apple purée (apple sauce)
2 large eggs, separated
A squeeze of lemon juice
Grated lemon peel

Tip the blancmange powder into a 1.75 litre/3 pt/7½ cup bowl. Mix smoothly with 60 ml/4 tbsp of the measured milk. Pour the remaining milk into a basin. Heat, uncovered, on Full for 4 minutes. Blend into the blancmange mixture. Add the sugar and stir thoroughly. Cook, uncovered, on Full for about 2½ minutes, beating every minute, until smooth and thickened. Whisk in the apple purée and egg yolks. Cover and allow to cool to lukewarm. Beat together the egg whites and lemon juice to stiff peaks. Whisk one-third into the blancmange mixture, then gently fold in the remainder with a large metal spoon.

Spoon into four dishes or glasses. Cover and chill for several hours. Sprinkle each lightly with lemon peel before serving.

Apricot Snow

Serves 4

Prepare as for Apple Snow, but substitute apricot purée (sauce) for the apple purée.

Lemon Meringue Spiced Pears

Serves 6

Altogether a surprise package.

75 g/3 oz/1/3 cup light soft brown sugar

300 ml/½ pt/1¼ cups water

60 ml/4 tbsp dry white wine

5 cm/2 inch piece cinnamon stick

4 whole cloves

6 firm dessert pears

1 packet lemon meringue filling mix

150 ml/¼ pt/2/3 cup milk, at kitchen temperature

Finely grated peel of 1 small lemon

Basil leaves, to decorate

Put the sugar, water, wine, cinnamon stick and cloves in a 1.75 litre/3 pt/7½ cup dish. Heat, uncovered, on Full for 3 minutes. Set aside. Peel the pears, leaving the stalks in place. Arrange upright in the dish and baste with the spicy syrup mixture. Slide the dish into a roasting bag and tie up with string. Cook on Full for 7 minutes. Remove from the microwave and take the dish from the bag. Carefully strain the syrup into a measuring jug. Stir in the lemon filling mix. Cover with saucer and cook on Full for 2–3 minutes, whisking every 30 seconds, until the mixture comes to the boil. Allow to cool for 5 minutes. Whisk in the milk and lemon peel. Cover and chill both the pears and the lemon sauce for several hours. Before serving, coat the pears with about half the sauce and decorate with basil leaves. Pour the remainder into a jug and pass separately.

Finnish Cranberry Whip

Serves 6

225 g/8 oz cranberries, thawed if frozen

150 ml/¼ pt/2/3 cup water

175 g/6 oz/¾ cup caster (superfine) sugar

5 ml/1 tsp finely grated lemon peel

150 ml/¼ pt/2/3 cup whipping cream

150 ml/¼ pt/2/3 cup double (heavy) cream

2 large egg whites

Put the cranberries, water, sugar and lemon peel in a 1.25 litre/2¼ pt/5½ cup dish. Cover with a plate and cook on Full for 8½ minutes, stirring twice and crushing the fruit against the side of the dish. Allow to cool completely. Whip the creams together until thick. Beat the egg whites to stiff peaks. Fold the cream and egg whites alternately into the cranberries. Transfer to six individual dishes. Chill lightly before serving.

Cranberry and Orange Whip

Serves 6

Prepare as for Finnish Cranberry Whip, but add 10 ml/2 tsp grated orange peel with the lemon peel.

Kissel

Serves 4

Russia's answer to blancmange, made from fruits growing wild in the countryside around country dachas or wooden holiday homes.

450 g/1 lb mixed soft berry fruits

60 ml/4 tbsp red wine, apple juice or water

75 g/3 oz/1/3 cup caster (superfine) sugar

5 ml/1 tsp vanilla essence (extract)

Peel of 1 lemon, cut into strips

15 ml/1 tbsp cornflour (cornstarch) or potato flour

30 ml/2 tbsp cold water

Single (light) cream or Home-made Yoghurt, to serve

Purée the fruit in a blender or food processor. Sieve to remove the seeds. Pour the wine, juice or water into a mixing bowl. Add the sugar, vanilla and lemon strips. Cover with a plate and cook on Full for 3½ minutes, stirring twice to ensure the sugar has dissolved. Add the berry purée. Cover as before and cook on Full for 2 minutes. Strain into a clean bowl. Blend the cornflour or potato flour smoothly with the water. Add to the fruit mixture. Cook, uncovered, on Full for 2–3 minutes, stirring three times, until thickened. Allow to cool slightly. Transfer to four dessert dishes, then cover and chill for several hours. Float cream or yoghurt over the top of each before serving.

Home-made Yoghurt

Makes about 900 ml/1½ pt/3¾ cups

900 ml/1½ pts/3¾ cups full-cream milk

60 ml/4 tbsp skimmed milk powder (non-fat dry milk)

150 ml/¼ pt/2/3 cup plain yoghurt

Pour the milk into a bowl. Heat, uncovered, on Defrost for about 4–5 minutes until lukewarm but not hot. Whisk in the skimmed milk and yoghurt. Cover. Leave to stand in a warm place for 12 hours until set – a linen cupboard is ideal. Store in the refrigerator when cold.

Apricot Pots

Serves 8

350 g/12 oz/2 cups dried apricot halves

600 ml/1 pt/2½ cups boiling water

30 ml/2 tbsp orange flower water

60 ml/4 tbsp icing (confectioners') sugar, sifted

225 g/8 oz/1 cup thick Greek-style plain yoghurt

Raspberry Coulis

Thoroughly wash the apricots, then soak in boiling water, covered with a plate, for at least 6 hours. Drain and transfer to a bowl. Add the measured boiling water. Cover with clingfilm (plastic wrap) and slit it twice to allow steam to escape. Cook on Defrost for 25–30 minutes, turning the bowl three times. Remove from the microwave and allow to cool to lukewarm. Tip into a food processor with the orange flower water and sugar and run the machine until the mixture forms a fairly smooth purée. Combine with the yoghurt and spoon evenly into eight ramekin dishes (custard cups). Cover and chill. Before serving, cover each with the coulis.

Prune Pots

Serves 8

350 g/12 oz dried stoned (pitted) prunes

600 ml/1 pt/2½ cups boiling water

30 ml/2 tbsp orange flower water

60 ml/4 tbsp icing (confectioners') sugar, sifted

30–45 ml/2–3 tbsp Armagnac

225 g/8 oz/1 cup thick Greek-style plain yoghurt

Chopped pecan nuts and demerara sugar, to serve

Thoroughly wash the prunes, then soak in boiling water, covered with plate, for at least 6 hours. Drain and transfer to a bowl. Add the measured boiling water. Cover with clingfilm (plastic wrap) and slit it twice to allow steam to escape. Cook on Defrost for 25–30 minutes, turning the bowl three times. Remove from the microwave and allow to cool to lukewarm. Tip the drained prunes, orange flower water, sugar and Armagnac into a food processor and run the machine until the mixture forms a fairly smooth purée. Combine with the yoghurt and spoon evenly into eight ramekin dishes (custard cups). Cover and chill. Before serving, sprinkle each with pecan nuts and demerara sugar.

Cherries Jubilee

Serves 6

One of North America's prize specimens and a show-off designed to impress.

400 g/14 oz/1 large can black cherry fruit filling
30 ml/2 tbsp cold water
30 ml/2 tbsp Kirsch or brandy
Vanilla ice cream

Put the fruit filling in a bowl and stir in the water. Heat, uncovered, on Defrost for 3 minutes. Stir round. Spread evenly into a shallow serving dish. In a separate dish, warm the spirit, uncovered, on Defrost for 45 seconds. Pour over the cherries and carefully ignite. Serve immediately over scoops of ice cream.

Fruits of the Forest Jubilee

Serves 6

Prepare as for Cherries Jubilee, but substitute apple and blackberry fruit filling for black cherry and strawberry ice cream for vanilla.

Dutch Chocolate Sundaes

Serves 4

90 ml/6 tbsp advocaat

75 ml/5 tbsp single (light) cream

2 small bananas, thinly sliced

Vanilla or chocolate ice cream

1 chocolate flake bar, crushed

Pour the advocaat into a dish and stir in the cream. Add the bananas. Heat, uncovered, on Defrost for 3 minutes. Mix gently. Spoon over scoops of ice cream in sundae dishes or dessert glasses and sprinkle with the chocolate flake. Eat straight away.

Cream Liqueur Sundaes

Serves 4

Prepare as for Dutch Chocolate Sundaes, but substitute any cream liqueur, quantity to taste, for the advocaat.

Grape and Raspberry Jelly

Serves 4

1 packet raspberry jelly (jello)

225 g/8 oz mixed black and green seedless grapes, rinsed and drained

Wafer biscuits (cookies), to serve

Snip the jelly into cubes with kitchen scissors and put in a measuring cup with 60 ml/4 tbsp cold water. Melt, uncovered, on Defrost for 2–2½ minutes. Make up to 450 ml/¾ pt/2 cups with cold water. Cover and chill until just beginning to thicken and set – it must not be at all runny. Fold the grapes into the thickened jelly with a spoon. Divide equally between four dessert dishes or stemmed glasses. Cover loosely with kitchen paper and chill until set. Serve with wafer biscuits.

Mandarin and Lemon Jelly

Serves 4

Prepare as for Grape and Raspberry Jelly, but substitute lemon jelly (jello) for the raspberry and peeled fresh mandarin, clementine or satsuma segments, halved, for the grapes.

Black Cherry Rice Cream

Serves 4

1 packet black cherry jelly (jello)

400 g/14 oz/1 large can rice pudding

75 ml/5 tbsp single (light) cream

30 ml/2 tbsp black cherry jam (conserve)

Snip the jelly into cubes with kitchen scissors and put in a measuring cup. Melt, uncovered, on Defrost for 2–2½ minutes. Fold in the rice pudding and cream, whisking gently without beating. Make up to 600 ml/1 pt/2½ cups with cold water. Cover lightly and chill until just beginning to thicken and set, stirring frequently. Divide equally between four sundae glasses and allow to set completely. Top each with 7.5 ml/1½ tsp jam before serving.

Banana Splits

Serves 4

The return of something special after a long time away.

Peel 4 large bananas, then halve each lengthways. Arrange on four plates. Put 2 scoops of vanilla ice cream in between each to make a 'sandwich', then top with any of the hot chocolate sauce recipes. Pipe or spoon on softly whipped cream and serve straight away.

Spicy Prune Froth

Serves 4

450 ml/¾ pt/2 cups prune juice

15 ml/1 tbsp powdered gelatine

8 cm/3 in piece cinnamon stick

2 star anise

30 ml/2 tbsp fine-shred orange marmalade

2 large egg whites

A pinch of salt

30 ml/2 tbsp whipped cream

Ground cinnamon

Pour 45 ml/3 tbsp of the prune juice into a small bowl. Add the gelatine and stir round. Stand for 5 minutes to soften. Melt, uncovered, on Defrost for 2–2½ minutes. Set aside. Pour the remaining prune juice into a large jug and add the cinnamon stick, star anise and marmalade. Heat, uncovered, on Full for 6 minutes or until the liquid just begins to bubble. Gently beat in the dissolved gelatine. Strain into a clean bowl. Cover with a plate and allow to cool, then chill until just beginning to thicken and set. Whisk the egg whites and salt until stiff. Beat one-third into the part-set prune jelly, then fold in the remaining whites thoroughly with large metal spoon or spatula. Spoon into four glass dishes, cover loosely and allow to set for several hours in the refrigerator. Before serving, decorate each with cream and dust with cinnamon.

Chilled Oranges with Hot Chocolate Peppermint Sauce

Serves 4

4 large oranges, peeled and very thinly sliced
Hot Chocolate Peppermint Sauce
Mint sprigs

Peel and very thinly slice the oranges, ensuring any pips (pits) are removed. Arrange on four side plates, then cover and chill until almost icy. Immediately before serving, drizzle the sauce over each, then garnish with mint sprigs.

Summer Fruit Mould

Serves 4

A sort of summer pudding in an instant. It is markedly sweet-sour and benefits from a drizzle of custard or sweetened cream.

500 g/1 lb 2 oz frozen mixed summer fruits
1 packet raspberry jelly (jello)

Tip the fruit into a bowl. Cover with a plate and thaw on Defrost for 7–8 minutes. Remove from the microwave. Snip the jelly into cubes and put in a bowl or jug. Melt, uncovered, on Defrost for 2½ minutes. Stir into the fruits. Chill until just beginning to thicken and set, stirring frequently so that the fruit stays suspended in the jelly. Transfer to a wetted mould or basin and cover. Chill until firm and completely set. Invert on to a plate and serve.

Watermelon and Apricot Chill with Frosted Grapes

Serves 4

150 ml/¼ pt/2/3 cup sweet white wine

150 ml/¼ pt/2/3 cup white grape juice

Peel of 1 lime, cut into narrow strips

175 g/6 oz/1 cup dried apricots, well washed and cut into strips

5 ml/1 tsp vanilla essence (extract)

2.5 ml/½ tsp almond essence (extract)

1 large wedge red watermelon

4 clusters black seedless grapes

1 small egg white, lightly beaten

Caster (superfine) sugar

Pour the wine and grape juice into a 1.25 litre/2¼ pt/5½ cup bowl. Add half the lime peel. Heat, uncovered, on Full for 4 minutes. Add the apricot strips. Cook, uncovered, on Full for 2 minutes. Stir in the vanilla and almond essence (extract). Cover and allow to cool. Thoroughly chill when cold. Slice the watermelon flesh away from its skin and remove all the black seeds. Cut the flesh into small cubes. Set aside. Wash and dry the grapes but leave attached to their stalks. Dip them in egg white to cover, then coat thickly with caster sugar. Leave to dry and set for at least an hour. Add the melon to the apricot mixture and transfer to four glass dessert dishes. Top each with a bunch of frosted grapes and the remaining lime peel, cut into narrow strips.

Rhubarb and Mandarin Cups

Serves 6

450 g/1 lb rhubarb, trimmed and chopped

300 gl/11 oz/1 large can mandarin oranges in syrup

60 ml/4 tbsp granulated sugar

5 ml/1 tsp finely grated orange peel

Raspberry or strawberry sorbet

Put the rhubarb in a 1.25 litre/2¼ pt/5½ cup dish with 30 ml/2 tbsp syrup from the mandarins and all the sugar. Cover with a plate and cook on Full for 7–9 minutes until the rhubarb is tender. Uncover and stir in the drained mandarins and orange peel. Cover and cool, then chill for several hours. Spoon into six glasses over scoops of sorbet and eat straight away.

Rhubarb and Mandarin Cups with Ginger Cream

Serves 6

450 g/1 lb rhubarb, trimmed and chopped

300 gl/11 oz/1 large can mandarin oranges in syrup

60 ml/4 tbsp granulated sugar

5 ml/1 tsp finely grated orange peel

5 ml/1 tsp ginger jam (conserve)

90 ml/6 tbsp double (heavy) cream, whipped

Vanilla ice cream

Put the rhubarb in a 1.25 litre/2¼ pt/5½ cup dish with 30 ml/2 tbsp syrup from the mandarins and all the sugar. Cover with a plate and cook on Full for 7–9 minutes until the rhubarb is tender. Uncover and stir in the drained mandarins and orange peel. Cover and cool, then chill for several hours. Mix the jam lightly into the cream. Spoon the rhubarb and mandarin mixture into six glasses over scoops of ice cream and top each with 25 ml/1½ tbsp of the ginger cream. Eat straight away.

Chocolate Strawberries on Pineapple Sorbet

Serves 4

175 g/6 oz plain (semi-sweet) chocolate

15 g/½ oz/1 tbsp unsalted (sweet) butter

16–20 large unhulled strawberries, washed and dried

Pineapple sorbet

Break up the chocolate and place in a dish with the butter. Melt, uncovered, on Defrost for about 3½ minutes. If the chocolate stays on the firm side, give it 10-second bursts on Defrost until just runny – do not overheat or the chocolate will become granular. Holding each strawberry by its green hull and stalk, swirl it round in the chocolate until three-quarters covered. Stand on a baking tray lined with greaseproof (waxed) paper and leave in the cool to set. To serve, put scoops of sorbet into four glass dessert dishes and top each with the strawberries.

Danish Apple 'Cake'

Serves 4–6

An old friend from Denmark, and a distinguished and handsome-looking sundae – not remotely like a cake.

750 g/1½ lb cooking (tart) apples, peeled and sliced
45 ml/3 tbsp boiling water
90 ml/6 tbsp caster (superfine) sugar
125 g/4 oz/½ cup butter
100 g/3½ oz/1¾ cups fresh white breadcrumbs
30 ml/2 tbsp light soft brown sugar
150 ml/¼ pt/2/3 cup double (heavy) cream
15 ml/1 tbsp milk
20–60 ml/4–6 tsp red jam (conserve)

Put the apple slices in a 1.75 litre/3 pt/7½ cup dish with the boiling water. Cover with a plate and cook on Full for 7–8 minutes until very soft. Beat to a pulp, then stir in the caster sugar. Set aside. Melt the butter in a frying pan (skillet). Add the breadcrumbs and fry (sauté) conventionally until lightly browned. Stir in the brown sugar. Allow to cool. Fill four to six sundae or other tall glasses with alternate layers of apples and crumbs, ending with crumbs. Whip the cream and milk until softly stiff. Pile on top of each portion, then add 5 ml/1 tsp of jam to each.

Peasant Girl with Veil

Serves 4–6

A variation on Danish Apple Cake, this is also Danish but uses 5 slices of crumbled rye bread instead of white breadcrumbs. Otherwise the ingredients and method are the same.

Imperial Rice

Serves 6–8

An old French traditional recipe, simplified by the use of store cupboard ingredients.

400 g/14 oz/1 large can rice pudding

400–450 g/14–16 oz/1 large can custard

25 ml/1½ tbsp powdered gelatine

125 ml/4 fl oz/½ cup cold water

60 ml/4 tbsp smooth apricot jam (conserve)

5 ml/1 tsp vanilla essence (extract)

2.5 ml/½ tsp almond essence (extract)

30 ml/2 tbsp assorted coloured glacé (candied) cherries, coarsely chopped

Combine the rice pudding and custard in a 2 litre/3½ pt/8½ cup bowl. Put the gelatine into a small bowl and stir in half the water. Heat, uncovered, on Defrost for 1¾–2 minutes until melted and the liquid is clear. Add the remaining water. Stir gently into the rice and custard mixture. Spoon the jam into the emptied small bowl. Warm, uncovered, on Defrost for 1–1½ minutes. Stir into the rice mixture with the vanilla and almond essence (extract). Cover and chill until just on the point of setting. Stir in the cherries. Rinse a 1.5 litre/2½ pt/6 cup jelly (jello) mould with cold water, then fill with the rice mixture. Cover and chill until firm and set. Turn out and serve with any of the fruit sauces.

Children's Fruity Mousse

Serves 4–6

An easy and economical sweet that reached its heyday in the fifties.

1 packet strawberry jelly (jello)

300 ml/½ pt/1¼ cups cold water

175 ml/6 fl oz/1 small can full-cream evaporated milk, chilled overnight in the refrigerator

30 ml/2 tbsp fresh or bottled lemon juice

Whipped cream and fruit, to decorate (optional)

Snip the jelly into cubes and put in a measuring jug. Cover with a plate and melt on Defrost for 2–2½ minutes. Gradually stir in the water. Keep covered and leave in the cool until just beginning to thicken. Beat the chilled evaporated milk until light and frothy. Add the lemon juice, a little at a time, and continue whisking until the milk thickens to the consistency of whipped cream. Whisk in the still liquid jelly lightly but smoothly. Transfer to four to six small dishes and chill until set. Decorate with cream and/or canned or fresh fruit, if liked.

Raspberry and Blackcurrant Mousse

Serves 4

A more sophisticated version of Children's Fruity Mousse that can confidently be served to adults.

1 packet raspberry jelly (jello)
150 ml/¼ pt/2/3 cup cold water
150 ml/¼ pt/2/3 cup raspberry purée made from fresh or frozen raspberries
175 ml/6 fl oz/1 small can full-cream evaporated milk, chilled overnight in the refrigerator
30 ml/2 tbsp fresh or bottled lemon juice
Whipped cream and fresh blackcurrants, to decorate

Snip the jelly into cubes and put in a measuring jug. Cover with a plate and melt on Defrost for 2–2½ minutes. Gradually stir in the water and raspberry purée. Keep covered and leave in the cool until just beginning to thicken. Beat the chilled evaporated milk until light and frothy. Add the lemon juice, a little at a time, and continue whisking until the milk thickens to the consistency of whipped cream. Whisk in the still liquid jelly lightly but smoothly. Swirl into four wine glasses and chill until set. Decorate with cream and blackcurrants.

Welsh Rarebit

Serves 2

125 g/4 oz/1 cup Cheddar cheese, grated
5 ml/1 tsp mustard powder
5 ml/1 tsp cornflour (cornstarch)
1 egg yolk
10 ml/2 tsp milk
Salt and freshly ground black pepper
2 large slices freshly made toast
Paprika

Mix the cheese with the mustard, cornflour, egg yolk and milk. Season to taste. Spread over the toast. Transfer to individual plates. Cook one at a time, uncovered, on Full for 1 minute. Sprinkle lightly with paprika and eat straight away.

Mixed Cheese Rarebit

Serves 2

Prepare as for Welsh Rarebit, but substitute 50 g/2 oz/½ cup crumbled Stilton cheese for half the Cheddar.

Buck Rarebit

Serves 2

Prepare as for Welsh Rarebit, but top each slice with a fried (sautéed) egg, cooked either in the microwave or conventionally.

Bacon Rarebit

Serves 2

Put 4 streaky bacon rashers (slices) on a plate and cover with kitchen paper. Cook on Full for 2½ minutes. Prepare the Welsh Rarebit and top each slice with 2 bacon rashers.

Beer Rarebit

Serves 4

Slightly more ornate, this is a substantial snack for midday or the evening.

25 g/1 oz/2 tbsp butter or margarine, at kitchen temperature

5 ml/1 tsp mild made mustard

2.5 ml/½ tsp Worcestershire sauce

5 ml/1 tsp tomato ketchup (catsup)

225 g/8 oz/2 cups Cheddar cheese, grated

45 ml/3 tbsp dark ale

4 slices freshly made toast

1 large tomato, sliced

Chopped parsley

Bacon and fried (sautéed) or poached eggs (optional), to serve

Combine the butter or margarine with the mustard, Worcestershire sauce, ketchup, cheese and ale. Spread equal amounts over the toast. Transfer to four individual plates. Cook, uncovered one at a time, on Full for 1 minute. Add the tomato slices and a sprinkling of parsley. If liked, top with bacon and/or eggs.

Open-topped Hungarian Salami Sandwiches

Serves 4

These are based on a recipe found in a leaflet at a Hungarian trade fair held in London. The subtle smokiness of the salami gives the sandwiches a continental flair.

4 spring onions (scallions), finely chopped
75 g/3 oz Hungarian salami, rinded and finely chopped
175 g/6 oz/1½ cups Emmental cheese, finely grated
2 egg yolks
4 large slices freshly made toast
Pickled cucumber slices, to garnish

Put the onions and salami in a bowl and combine with the cheese and egg yolks. Spread over the toast. Cook one at a time, uncovered, on Full for 1–1½ minutes until the cheese melts. Serve straight away.

Granola

Makes about 750 g/1½ lb/6 cups

Like dry and sweet muesli with a distinctive crackle and a crunch, this is an import from North America where it is eaten as a breakfast cereal with milk or as a nibble instead of biscuits (cookies). Diet food it isn't, but it can be enjoyed as an occasional weekend treat.

125 g/4 oz/½ cup butter or margarine

90 ml/6 tbsp golden (light corn) syrup

250 g/9 oz/2¼ cups porridge oats

45 ml/3 tbsp coarse bran

100 g/3½ oz/scant ½ cup light soft brown sugar

75 g/3 oz/¾ cup chopped nuts

100 g/3½ oz/2/3 cup raisins

Put the butter or margarine in a 25 cm/10 in diameter casserole dish (Dutch oven). Add the syrup. Melt, uncovered, on Defrost for 4 minutes. Mix in all the remaining ingredients except the raisins. Cook, uncovered, on Full for 9½ minutes, stirring four or five times, until the granola is lightly browned. Add the raisins and mix in thoroughly. Allow to stand until cold and crisp, then break up with a fork until crumbly. Store in an airtight container.

Honey Granola

Makes about 750 g/1½ lb/6 cups

Prepare as for Granola, but substitute clear honey for the syrup.

Porridge

For 1 portion: put 25 g/1 oz/¼ cup porridge oats in a cereal bowl. Add 150 ml/¼ pt/2/3 cup cold milk or water and a pinch of salt. Cook, uncovered, on Full for 1¾–2 minutes, stirring twice. Allow to stand for 1½ minutes before eating.

For 2 portions in 2 bowls: prepare as for 1 portion, but cook on Full for 3–3½ minutes.

For 3 portions in 3 bowls: prepare as for 1 portion, but cook on Full for 3½ –4 minutes.

Bacon

Bacon reacts well to microwave cooking and shrinks less than if grilled (broiled) or fried (sautéed) conventionally. Place the rasher or rashers (slices) in a single layer on a plate and cover lightly with kitchen paper to prevent spluttering and soiling the oven. The cooking time needed will vary according to the type and thickness of the bacon, but this is a general guide:

1 rasher: cook on Full for 45–60 seconds

2 rashers: cook on Full for 1½–1¾ minutes

3 rashers: cook on Full for 2–2¼ minutes

4 rashers: cook on Full for 2½–2¾ minutes

5 rashers: cook on Full for 3–3½ minutes

6 rashers: cook on Full for 4–4½ minutes

Drain the bacon on clean kitchen paper after cooking.

Basic White Sauce

Serves 4

The multi-purpose and versatile coating sauce known and appreciated internationally for its smooth and velvety texture and glossy appearance.

300 ml/½ pt/1¼ cups milk

25 g/1 oz/2 tbsp butter or margarine

25 g/1 oz/¼ cup plain (all-purpose) flour

Salt and freshly ground black pepper or caster (superfine) sugar

Pour the milk into a jug and warm, uncovered, on Full for 2 minutes. Put the butter or margarine in a 900 ml/1½ pt/3¾ cup bowl. Melt, uncovered, on Defrost for 1 minute. Stir in the flour to form a roux. Heat, uncovered, on Full for 30 seconds. Remove from the microwave and gradually blend in the warm milk. Cook, uncovered, on Full for 3–4 minutes, beating every minute for maximum smoothness, until the sauce comes to the boil and thickens. Season to taste with salt and pepper for a savoury sauce and caster sugar for a sweet one.

Béchamel Sauce

Serves 4

This the aristocratic version of Basic White Sauce, named after a steward of Louis XIV. It is important in the great kitchens of the western world and is deceptively easy to make. Use only for savoury dishes.

300 ml/½ pt/1¼ cups milk
1 bouquet garni sachet
1 bay leaf
1 small onion, peeled and quartered
2 large parsley sprigs
1.5 ml/¼ tsp grated nutmeg
25 g/1 oz/2 tbsp butter or margarine
25 g/1 oz/¼ cup plain (all-purpose) flour
Salt and freshly ground black pepper

Pour the milk into a 900 ml/1½ pt/3¾ cup jug. Add the bouquet garni, bay leaf, onion, parsley and nutmeg. Cover with a saucer and bring just up to the boil, allowing 5–6 minutes on Defrost. Remove from the microwave, keep covered, and allow to cool to lukewarm. Strain. Put the butter or margarine in a 900 ml/1½ pt/3¾ cup bowl. Melt, uncovered, on Defrost for 1 minute. Stir in the flour to form a roux. Heat, uncovered, on Full for 30 seconds. Remove from the microwave and gradually blend in the flavoured milk. Cook, uncovered, on Full for 3–4 minutes, beating every minute for maximum smoothness, until the sauce comes to the boil and thickens. Season to taste with salt and pepper.

Caper Sauce

Serves 4

For skate, herring, mackerel and lamb.

Prepare as for Basic White Sauce, but add 20 ml/4 tsp drained and chopped capers half-way through the cooking time.

Cheese Sauce

Serves 4

For bacon and gammon, fish, poultry and vegetables.

Prepare as for Basic White Sauce, but add 50–75 g/2–3 oz/½–¾ cup grated hard cheese and 5 ml/1 tsp made mustard half-way through the cooking time.

Mornay Sauce

Serves 4

A close relation of Cheese Sauce, also for bacon and gammon, fish, poultry and vegetables.

Prepare as for Basic White Sauce, but use milk seasoned with salt and freshly ground black pepper and add 50–75 g/2–3 oz/½–¾ cup grated Gruyère (Swiss) cheese half-way through the cooking time.

Egg Sauce

Serves 4

Also known as Dutch Egg Sauce or Mock Hollandaise. For fish and poultry.

Prepare as for Basic White Sauce, but add 2 chopped hard-boiled (hard-cooked) eggs with the seasoning.

Mushroom Sauce

Serves 4

For fish and poultry and egg dishes such as omelettes.

Heat 50 g/2 oz/½ cup thinly sliced mushrooms with 10 ml/2 tsp butter on Full for 1½ minutes. Mix into the prepared Basic White Sauce half-way through the cooking time. Season to taste with ground nutmeg.

Mustard Sauce

Serves 4

Serve with pork and gammon, offal and oily fish such as mackerel and herring.

Prepare as for Basic White Sauce, but add 10–15 ml/2–3 tsp English made mustard and 10 ml/2 tsp lemon juice with the seasoning.

Onion Sauce

Serves 4

For grilled (broiled) and roast lamb.

Chop 1 onion and put into a small dish with 25 ml/1½ tbsp cold water and 1.5 ml/¼ tsp salt. Cover with clingfilm (plastic wrap) and slit it twice to allow steam to escape. Cook on Full for 4–5 minutes until soft. Mix into the prepared Basic White Sauce.

Parsley Sauce

Serves 4

For fish, vegetables, poultry and boiled bacon.

Prepare as for Basic White Sauce, but add 45–60 ml/3–4 tbsp chopped parsley with the seasoning.

Watercress Sauce

Serves 4

For fish and poultry.

Prepare as for Basic White Sauce, but add 45–60 ml/3–4 tbsp chopped watercress with the seasoning.

Pouring Sauce

Serves 4

Prepare as for Basic White Sauce, but reduce the flour to 15 g/½ oz/1 tbsp. Either season with salt and pepper and use as a white 'gravy', or sweeten with sugar and serve over steamed or baked pudding.

All-in-one Sauce

Serves 4

A high-speed version of Basic White Sauce.

25 g/1 oz/¼ cup plain (all-purpose) flour
300 ml/½ pt/1¼ cups milk
25 g/1 oz/2 tbsp butter or margarine
Salt and freshly ground black pepper or caster (superfine) sugar

Whisk the flour into the milk in a bowl, then add the butter or margarine. Cook, uncovered, on Full for 6–6½ minutes, whisking four or five times, until thick and smooth. Flavour to taste.

Hollandaise Sauce

Serves 6–8

One of the great sauces of our time, Hollandaise made conventionally needs skill and culinary artistry. In the microwave it behaves as though you were a chef of unquestionable brilliance. Use it with poached salmon and trout, broccoli and cauliflower, with artichokes and asparagus.

125 g/4 oz/½ cup slightly salted butter
15 ml/1 tbsp lemon juice, strained
2 egg yolks
Salt and freshly ground black pepper
A pinch of caster (superfine) sugar

Put the butter in a 900 ml/1½ pt/3¾ cup jug or dish. Melt, uncovered, on Full for 1½ minutes until hot and bubbling. Add the lemon juice and egg yolks and whisk thoroughly. Return to the microwave and cook on Full for 30 seconds. Stir briskly. The sauce is ready when it is as thick as cold custard and clings to the whisk; if not, cook for a further 15 seconds. Season to taste, then add the sugar to counteract the sharpness of the lemon juice. Serve warm. Watch the cooking time very carefully because Hollandaise that refuses to thicken and looks curdled has been overcooked. One remedy is to beat in 30–45 ml/2–3 tbsp very cold water; a second is to beat in 30 ml/2 tbsp double (heavy) cream; a third is to beat the curdled sauce into a fresh egg yolk and return to the microwave for a few seconds until thick and smooth.

Short-cut Béarnaise Sauce

Serves 6–8

Recommended for steaks and rare roast beef.

Prepare as for Hollandaise Sauce, but substitute wine vinegar for the lemon juice and add 2.5 ml/½ tsp dried tarragon with the seasoning and sugar.

Maltese Sauce

Serves 6–8

For freshwater fish and poultry.

Prepare as for Hollandaise Sauce, but stir in 5 ml/1 tsp very finely grated orange peel with the seasoning and sugar.

Mayonnaise Sauce

Makes 600 ml/1 pt/2½ cups

Because of the current disquiet associated with eating raw egg yolk, the eggs in this mayonnaise are blended with very hot liquid, which is equivalent to being partially cooked and is therefore safer than standard home-made mayonnaise based on entirely raw yolks. The texture is thinner than traditional mayonnaise but, when cold, is thick enough to coat foods satisfactorily. It is also excellent as a mixer sauce with coleslaw and potato salad.

600 ml/1 pt/2½ cups sunflower or safflower oil
30 ml/2 tbsp lemon juice
15 ml/1 tbsp wine or cider vinegar
2.5 ml/½ tsp caster (superfine) sugar
15–20 ml/3–4 tsp salt
5 ml/1 tsp made mustard
2 large eggs

Spoon 75 ml/5 tbsp of the oil into a small bowl. Add the lemon juice, vinegar, sugar, salt and mustard. Heat, uncovered, on Defrost for 3–4 minutes until very hot. Break the eggs into a blender and add the hot oil mixture. Run the machine until smooth. With the machine still running but the lid removed, add the remaining oil in a thin steady stream. Transfer to a bowl. Cover and chill until cold and thick. Keep refrigerated in screw-topped jar and use as required.

Cocktail Sauce

Makes 600 ml/1 pt/2½ cups

A classic for seafood.

Prepare as for Mayonnaise Sauce. After it has thickened, stir in 30 ml/2 tbsp tomato purée (paste), 10 ml/2 tsp horseradish, a dash of hot pepper sauce such as Tabasco and 5 ml/1 tsp Worcestershire sauce.

Louis Sauce

Makes 600 ml/1 pt/2½ cups

A sauce from San Francisco created in the early twentieth century by a chef called Louis Diat. It is specially for crab salad.

600 ml/1 pt/2½ cups sunflower or safflower oil

30 ml/2 tbsp lemon juice

15 ml/1 tbsp wine or cider vinegar

2.5 ml/½ tsp caster (superfine) sugar

15–20 ml/3–4 tsp salt

5 ml/1 tsp made mustard

2 large eggs

Chilli or hot pepper sauce

60 ml/4 tbsp whipping cream, softly whipped

¼ green (bell) pepper, seeded and finely chopped

15 ml/1 tbsp finely chopped spring onion (scallion)

Juice of ½ small lemon

Spoon 75 ml/5 tbsp of the oil into a small bowl. Add the lemon juice, vinegar, sugar, salt and mustard. Heat, uncovered, on Defrost for 3–4 minutes until very hot. Break the eggs into a blender and add the hot oil mixture. Run the machine until smooth. With the machine still running but the lid removed, add the remaining oil in a thin steady stream. Transfer to a bowl. Cover and chill until cold and thick. Stir in chilli or hot pepper sauce to make it gently hot, then add the cream, green pepper, spring onion and lemon juice. Keep refrigerated in a screw-topped jar and use as required.

Thousand Island Dressing

Makes 600 ml/1 pt/2½ cups

600 ml/1 pt/2½ cups sunflower or safflower oil

30 ml/2 tbsp lemon juice

15 ml/1 tbsp wine or cider vinegar

2.5 ml/½ tsp caster (superfine) sugar

15–20 ml/3–4 tsp salt

5 ml/1 tsp made mustard

2 large eggs

A dash of chilli or hot pepper sauce

1–2 hard-boiled (hard-cooked) eggs (pages 98–9), finely chopped

30–45 ml/2–3 tbsp tomato ketchup (catsup)

15 ml/1 tbsp finely chopped onion

15 ml/1 tbsp chopped parsley

30 ml/2 tbsp chopped stuffed olives (optional)

30 ml/2 tbsp whipped cream (optional)

Spoon 75 ml/5 tbsp of the oil into a small bowl. Add the lemon juice, vinegar, sugar, salt and mustard. Heat, uncovered, on Defrost for 3–4 minutes until very hot. Break the eggs into a blender and add the hot oil mixture. Run the machine until smooth. With the machine still running but the lid removed, add the remaining oil in a thin steady stream. Transfer to a bowl. Cover and chill until cold and thick. Stir in the chilli or hot pepper sauce, chopped eggs, tomato ketchup, onion, parsley and olives and cream, if using. Keep refrigerated in a screw-topped jar and use as required.

Green Sauce

Makes 600 ml/1 pt/2½ cups

Designed for fish.

Prepare as for Mayonnaise Sauce. After it has thickened, stir in 15 ml/1 tbsp chopped parsley, 15 ml/1 tbsp snipped chives and 15 ml/1 tbsp watercress. A little chopped tarragon may also be added.

Rémoulade Sauce

Makes 600 ml/1 pt/2½ cups

Superb with cold meats, beef in particular, and fish dishes.

Prepare as for Mayonnaise Sauce. After it has thickened, mix in 4 chopped anchovy fillets in oil, 5 ml/1 tsp French mustard, 5 ml/1 tsp chopped tarragon and 5 ml/1 tsp chopped parsley, 10 ml/2 tsp chopped gherkins (cornichons) and 10 ml/2 tsp chopped capers. A little chopped chervil may also be added.

Sauce Tartare

Makes 600 ml/1 pt/2½ cups

For fish.

Prepare as for Mayonnaise Sauce. After it has thickened, stir in 45 ml/3 tbsp chopped gherkins (cornichons), 30 ml/2 tbsp chopped parsley and 15 ml/1 tbsp finely chopped capers.

No-egg Mayonnaise-style Dressing

Serves 4

60 ml/4 tbsp cold water
90 ml/6 tbsp sunflower oil
1 oz/25 g/1/3 cup milk powder (non-fat dry milk)
2.5 ml/½ tsp salt
2.5 ml/½ tsp mustard powder
20 ml/4 tsp wine or cider vinegar
10 ml/2 tsp lemon juice
A pinch of sugar

Pour the water into a small bowl. Heat, uncovered, on Full for 1 minute until hot. Pour into blender or food processor and add all the remaining ingredients. Run the machine until smooth. Spoon into small bowl, cover and chill until cold. The dressing thickens up considerably if left overnight but can be thinned down to the desired consistency with warm water.

Mint Sauce

Serves 4–5

A very British sauce for roast lamb.

60 ml/4 tbsp finely chopped fresh mint leaves

60 ml/4 tbsp water

15 ml/1 tbsp caster (superfine) sugar

75 ml/5 tbsp malt vinegar

Salt and freshly ground black pepper

Put all the ingredients into a measuring cup. Heat, uncovered, on Full for 3 minutes. Serve cold.

Orange Sauce

serves 6–8

For cold meats and barbecued foods.

225 g/8 oz/1 cup redcurrant jelly (clear conserve)

Finely grated peel and juice of 1 orange

10 ml/2 tsp Grand Marnier

Put the redcurrant jelly with the orange peel and juice in a 1.25 litre/2¼ pt/5½ cup measuring jug. Heat, uncovered, on Defrost for 5–6 minutes, stirring three or four times, until the jelly melts. Allow the sauce to cool, then mix in the Grand Marnier. Serve cold.

Jellied Mixed Herb Sauce

Serves 8–10

For lamb.

450 ml/¾ pt/2 cups white grape or apple juice

15 ml/1 tbsp powdered gelatine

2.5 ml/½ tsp salt

30 ml/2 tbsp chopped mint

45 ml/3 tbsp snipped chives

40 ml/2½ tbsp chopped coriander (cilantro) leaves

Pour 45 ml/3 tbsp of the fruit juice into a 1.25 litre/2¼ pt/5½ cup bowl. Stir in the gelatine. Allow to stand for 5 minutes to soften. Melt, uncovered, on Defrost for 2–2½ minutes. Stir in the remaining juice with the salt. Cover when cold and chill until just beginning to thicken and set round the edge. Mix in all the remaining ingredients. Transfer to a small serving dish and chill until set completely. Spoon out on to plates to serve.

Jellied Herb Sauce with Lemon

Serves 8–10

For fish.

Prepare as for Jellied Mixed Herb Sauce, but substitute chopped parsley for the coriander (cilantro) and add 10 ml/2 tsp grated lemon rind with the other ingredients.

Salsa

Serves 6

A simple version of the trendy Mexican sauce-cum-condiment which can be used as a dip or eaten with Mexican-style food. It also adds a bit of character to roasts and grilled (broiled) foods, bland cheeses like Mozzarella and omelettes. Some salsas are left uncooked, but heating this rather chunky version has a mellowing effect on the flavours.

3 large tomatoes, blanched, skinned, seeded and chopped
1 sweet or Spanish onion, finely grated
1–2 whole green chillies, seeded and finely chopped
1–2 garlic cloves, crushed
30 ml/2 tbsp chopped coriander (cilantro) leaves
5–10 ml/1–2 tsp salt

Place the tomatoes in a 1.25 litre/2¼ pt/5½ cup bowl with the onion, chilli and garlic. Cover with a plate and heat on Full for 3 minutes. Allow to cool completely. Stir in the coriander and salt before serving.

Smooth Salsa

Serves 6

Prepare as for Salsa, but transfer the ingredients to a blender after cooking and work to a smooth purée before adding the coriander and salt.

Extra-hot Salsa

Serves 6

Prepare as for Salsa, but double or even treble the quantity of green chillies. Take care when eating.

Coriander Salsa

Serves 6

Prepare as for Salsa, but increase the quantity of coriander (cilantro) to 25 g/1 oz/¼ cup.

Apple Sauce

Serves 4

Obligatory for roast pork, duck and goose.

450 g/1 lb cooking (tart) apples, peeled, quartered, cored and thinly sliced

45 ml/3 tbsp boiling water

10–15 ml/2–3 tsp granulated sugar

10 ml/2 tsp butter or margarine

Put the apples in a 1.25 litre/2¼ pt/5½ cup bowl with the water. Cover with a plate and cook on Full for 7–8 minutes until soft and pulpy, stirring twice. Beat until smooth. Mix in the sugar and butter or margarine. Serve warm or cold.

Mrs Beeton's Brown Apple Sauce

Serves 4

Prepare as for Apple Sauce, but cook the apples with a thin gravy instead of water.

Gooseberry Sauce

Serves 4

An old English sauce, traditionally served with goose, duck and mackerel.

Prepare as for Apple Sauce, but substitute 225 g/8 oz/2 cups trimmed gooseberries for the apples and add 5 ml/1 tsp finely grated lemon peel with the other ingredients.

Salsa with Sweetcorn

Serves 4

For barbecued foods.

10 ml/2 tsp corn oil

3 spring onions (scallions), finely chopped

30 ml/2 tbsp finely chopped coriander (cilantro) leaves

1 canned red pimiento, drained and chopped

2 large beef tomatoes, blanched, skinned, seeded and chopped

175 g/6 oz/1½ cups frozen sweetcorn (corn), thawed

10 ml/2 tsp jalapeno sauce

10 ml/2 tsp fresh lime juice

5 ml/1 tsp salt

Pour the oil into a 1.25 litre/2¼ pt/5½ cup bowl. Add the onions, coriander and pimiento. Cook, uncovered, on Full for 2½ minutes, stirring once. Mix in the tomatoes and sweetcorn. Cover with a plate and heat on Full for 2 minutes. Allow to cool completely. Stir in the remaining ingredients.

Austrian Apple and Horseradish Sauce

Serves 6–8

An example of the unusual and the unexpected, a remarkable hot sauce for beef.

450 g/1 lb cooking (tart) apples, peeled, quartered, cored and thinly sliced

30 ml/2 tbsp boiling water

10 ml/2 tsp icing (confectioners') sugar, sifted

30 ml/2 tbsp blanched and finely chopped almonds

15–45 ml/1–3 tbsp finely grated fresh horseradish or 30–45 ml/2–3 tbsp creamed horseradish

2.5–5 ml/½–1 tsp salt

10 ml/2 tsp malt vinegar

Put the apples in a 1.25 litre/2¼ pt/5½ cup bowl with the water. Cover with a plate and cook on Full for 7–8 minutes until soft and pulpy, stirring twice. Stir in all the remaining ingredients. Cover as before and cook on Full for 1½ minutes. Serve hot.

Garlic Sauce

Serves 4–6

An extremely garlicky sauce from Italy, designed for tossing into hot pasta dishes.

45 ml/3 tbsp olive oil

50 g/2 oz/¼ cup butter

6 garlic cloves, crushed

30 ml/2 tbsp finely chopped parsley

2.5 ml/½ tsp dried basil

2.5–5 ml/½–1 tsp salt

Freshly ground black pepper, to taste

Put all the ingredients in a 600 ml/1 pt/2½ cup bowl. Cover with a plate and warm on Defrost for 3–4 minutes, stirring once. Toss with piping hot spaghetti or other pasta and eat straight away.

Apple and Horseradish Sauce

Serves 6–8

An apple sauce from Romania, to serve with chicken.

50 g/2 oz/¼ cup butter

2 large cooking (tart) apples, peeled and grated

50 g/2 oz/½ cup plain (all-purpose) flour

450 ml/¾ pt/2 cups hot chicken stock

5–10 ml/1–2 tsp grated horseradish or 10 ml/2 tsp horseradish sauce

Salt

150 ml/¼ pt/2/3 cup whipping cream, whipped until thick

Sifted icing (confectioners') sugar (optional)

Put the butter in a 1.5 litre/2½ pt/6 cup bowl and heat, uncovered, on Full for 1¼ minutes. Mix in the apples and cook, uncovered, on Full for 3 minutes, stirring once. Stir in the flour and cook on Full for 20 seconds. Gradually blend in the hot stock. Cook, uncovered, on Full for 4–5 minutes, whisking every minute, until smoothly thickened. Stir in the horseradish, season to taste with salt, then fold in the cream. If the sauce is too sour for personal taste, stir in a little icing sugar. Serve straight away.

Bread Sauce

Serves 6–8

A vintage tradition with poultry.

300 ml/½ pt/1¼ cups milk

1 bouquet garni sachet

1 bay leaf

1 small onion, peeled and quartered

2 large parsley sprigs

1.5 ml/¼ tsp grated nutmeg

65 g/2½ oz fresh white breadcrumbs from crustless bread

15–25 g/½–1 oz/1–2 tbsp butter or margarine

Salt and freshly ground black pepper

Pour the milk into a 900 ml/1½ pt/3¾ cup jug. Add the bouquet garni, bay leaf, onion, parsley and nutmeg. Cover with a saucer and bring just to the boil on Defrost, allowing about 5–6 minutes. Remove from the microwave, keep covered and allow to cool to lukewarm. Strain. Add the crumbs. Cook, uncovered, on Defrost until thickened, allowing about 4–6 minutes and stirring every minute. Mix in the butter or margarine and season to taste. Reheat, uncovered, on Defrost for 1 minute.

Brown Bread Sauce

Serves 6–8

Prepare as for Bread Sauce, but substitute fresh breadcrumbs from crustless brown bread in place of the white.

Cranberry Sauce

Serves 6–8

A sweet-sour, fruity winter sauce and a sparkling and brilliant accompaniment for poultry.

225 g/8 oz/2 cups cranberries, thawed if frozen
150 ml/¼ pt/2/3 cup water
175 g/6 oz/¾ cup granulated sugar
5 ml/1 tsp finely grated lemon peel

Put all the ingredients in a 1.25 litre/2¼ pt/5½ cup bowl. Cover with a plate and cook on Full for 8–8½ minutes, stirring twice and crushing the fruit against the side of the bowl, until the fruit is soft. Remove from the microwave, keep covered and serve when cold. Keep any leftovers refrigerated in a covered container.

Cranberry Wine Sauce

Serves 6–8

Prepare as for Cranberry Sauce, but substitute red wine for the water.

Cranberry Orange Sauce

Serves 6–8

Prepare as for Cranberry Sauce, but substitute orange juice for the water.

Cranberry and Apple Sauce

Serves 6–8

Prepare as for Cranberry Sauce, but substitute 1 sliced cooking (tart) apple for half the cranberries.

Cumberland Sauce

Serves 6

A full-bodied and typically English sauce for ham, pork and tongue.

5 ml/1 tsp mild made mustard

30 ml/2 tbsp light soft brown sugar

1.5 ml/¼ tsp ground ginger

A pinch of cayenne pepper

300 ml/½ pt/1¼ cups dry white wine or port

2 whole cloves

15 ml/1 tbsp cornflour (cornstarch)

30 ml/2 tbsp cold water

60 ml/4 tbsp redcurrant jelly (clear conserve)

5 ml/1 tsp grated orange peel

5 ml/1 tsp grated lemon peel

Juice of 1 small orange

Juice of 1 lemon

Put the mustard, sugar, ginger, cayenne, wine or port and cloves in a 1.25 litre/2¼ pt/5½ cup bowl and heat, uncovered, on Full for 6 minutes, stirring three times. Meanwhile, mix the cornflour smoothly with the cold water. Mix into the wine mixture with the remaining ingredients. Heat, uncovered, on Full for 4–6 minutes, stirring every minute, until the sauce is thickened and smooth and the jelly has melted. Serve hot.

Slovenian Wine Sauce

Serves 4–6

A vegetable purée and wine sauce enriched with cream. It goes particularly well with venison and pigeon.

50 g/2 oz/¼ cup salted butter

2 carrots, finely grated

30 ml/2 tbsp plain (all-purpose) flour

300 ml/½ pt/1¼ cups dry white wine

100 g/3½ oz mushrooms, sliced

1 small bay leaf

Salt and freshly ground black pepper

150 ml/¼ pt/2/3 cup soured (dairy sour) cream

Put the butter in a 1.25 litre/2¼ pt/5½ cup bowl and heat, uncovered, on Full for 1¼ minutes. Add the carrots. Two-thirds cover with a plate and cook on Full for 4 minutes, stirring twice. Mix in the flour, wine, mushrooms and bay leaf. Cover with a plate and cook on Full for 6–7 minutes until the ingredients are tender. Remove the bay leaf and season to taste. Transfer to a blender or food processor and work to a smooth purée. Return to the dish and stir in the cream. Reheat on Full for 1–1½ minutes.

Thin Gravy for Poultry

Serves 6

15 ml/1 tbsp cornflour (cornstarch)

25 ml/1½ tbsp cold water

1 chicken or vegetable stock cube or 7.5 ml/1½ tsp brown gravy powder

300 ml/½ pt/1¼ cups stock, including pan juices from a roast chicken or turkey

Salt and freshly ground black pepper

Blend the cornflour smoothly with the cold water in a 900 ml/1½ pt/3¾ cup bowl or jug. Crumble in the stock cube or mix in the gravy powder. Stir in the stock. Cook, uncovered, on Full for 4–6 minutes, stirring every minute, until the gravy has thickened slightly. Season to taste before serving.

Thick Gravy for Meat

Serves 6

Prepare as for Thin Gravy for Poultry, but use 30 ml/2 tbsp cornflour (cornstarch) mixed with 40 ml/2½ tbsp cold water.

Short-cut Oriental Sauce

Serves 6–8

A cross between an Indian and a Malaysian sauce, this is a marvellous vehicle for adding flavour to leftover cold meat and sausages.

300 ml/10 fl oz/1 can condensed cream of celery or mushroom soup
150 ml/¼ pt/2/3 cup boiling water
30 ml/2 tbsp tomato purée (paste)
15 ml/1 tbsp mild or hot curry paste
1 garlic clove, crushed
5 ml/1 tsp turmeric
30 ml/2 tbsp fruit chutney
15 ml/1 tbsp crunchy peanut butter
20 ml/4 tsp desiccated (shredded) coconut

Pour the soup into a 1.25 litre/2¼ pt/5½ cup bowl with half the water. Add all the remaining ingredients except the coconut. Cover with a plate and heat on Full for 4 minutes, whisking every minute. Allow to stand for 2 minutes. Whisk in the remaining water and the coconut. Reheat, uncovered on Full for 1 minute.

Indonesian-style Peanut Sauce

Serves 6–8

In the Far East this sauce is served over assorted cold cooked vegetables, rather like a salad dressing, but it can also be used as a punchy sauce for barbecued foods and meat on skewers.

15 ml/1 tbsp corn oil
2 onions, finely chopped
1 garlic clove, crushed
350 g/12 oz/1½ cups smooth peanut butter
10 ml/2 tsp light soft brown sugar
Juice of 1 small lemon
600 ml/1 pt/2½ cups boiling water
30 ml/2 tbsp brown table sauce
Salt and freshly ground black pepper

Pour the oil into a 1.25 litre/2¼ pt/5½ cup bowl. Heat on Full for 30 seconds. Stir in the onions and garlic. Cook, uncovered, on Full for 6 minutes, stirring three times. Mix in the peanut butter, sugar, lemon juice and half the water. Cook, uncovered, on Full for 2–3 minutes, stirring three times, until the sauce looks like porridge in texture. Remove from the microwave. Thin down the sauce by whisking in the remaining water, then season with the brown sauce and salt and pepper to taste.

Creole Sauce

Serves 6–8

A jazzy sauce from the Mississippi, featuring sunset colours and an abundance of Mediterranean produce. It goes well with eggs, poultry, beef and even makes a vegetarian topping for fluffy mashed potatoes or rice.

20 ml/4 tsp corn oil

1 large onion, grated

1 garlic clove, crushed

30 ml/2 tbsp stoned (pitted) green olives, chopped

½ small green (bell) pepper, seeded and finely chopped

50 g/2 oz mushrooms, chopped

1 small bay leaf

400 g/14 oz/1 large can chopped tomatoes

15 ml/1 tbsp chopped basil leaves

15 ml/1 tbsp chopped parsley

10 ml/2 tsp dark soft brown sugar

5 ml/1 tsp salt

5 ml/1 tsp Tabasco or any other hot pepper sauce

5 cm/2 inch strip lemon peel

Put the oil, onion and garlic in a 2 litre/3½ pt/8½ cup bowl. Cook, uncovered, on Full for 6 minutes, stirring three times. Mix in the olives, green pepper and mushrooms. Cook, uncovered, on Full for 2 minutes. Stir in all the remaining ingredients. Cover with clingfilm (plastic wrap) and slit it twice to allow steam to escape. Cook on Full for 6–7 minutes, turning the bowl three times, until the sauce is hot. Allow to stand for 2 minutes before using.

Quick Creole Sauce

Serves 4–6

30 ml/2 tbsp dried (bell) pepper flakes

300 ml/10 fl oz/1 can condensed tomato soup

75 ml/5 tbsp boiling water

2.5 ml/½ tsp dried oregano

5 ml/1 tsp light soft brown sugar

5 ml/1 tsp Worcestershire sauce

Cover the pepper flakes with boiling water and leave for 3 minutes. Drain thoroughly. Put the soup and measured boiling water in a 1.25 litre/2¼ pt/5½ cup dish and beat until smooth. Mix in the remaining ingredients. Heat, uncovered, on Full for 4–5 minutes, stirring three times, until very hot.

Newburg Sauce

Serves 4

Associated primarily with lobster, this grandiose sauce goes equally well with many other shellfish, crab in particular.

25 g/1 oz/2 tbsp butter

1 small onion, grated

30 ml/2 tbsp plain (all-purpose) flour

300 ml/½ pt/1¼ cups single (light) cream, heated to lukewarm

3 egg yolks

60 ml/4 tbsp dry sherry or white port

Salt and freshly ground black pepper

Melt the butter, uncovered, on Full for 1 minute in a 900 ml/1½ pt/3¾ cup bowl. Add the onion and cook, uncovered, on Full for 1 minute, stirring once. Stir in the flour and cook, uncovered, on Full for 1 minute. Gradually blend in the cream. Cook, uncovered, on Full for 4–4½ minutes, whisking every minute, until thickened and smooth. Beat together the egg yolks and sherry or port. Add to the sauce and season to taste. Return to the microwave and cook, uncovered, on Defrost for 1–1½ minutes. Whisk and serve.

Piquant Brown Sauce

Serves 4–6

Based on a classic French sauce, this is a cheat's version that turns up trumps for grilled (broiled) foods and roasts and old family friends like sausages, toad-in-the-hole and corned beef.

300 ml/10 fl oz/1 can condensed oxtail soup

75 ml/5 tbsp boiling water

15 ml/1 tbsp chopped coriander (cilantro) leaves

15 ml/1 tbsp chopped parsley

15 ml/1 tbsp chopped capers

15 ml/1 tbsp chopped gherkins (cornichons)

2.5 ml/½ tsp dried mixed herbs

15 ml/1 tbsp brown table sauce

15 ml/1 tbsp port

Salt and freshly ground black pepper

Put all the ingredients in a 1.25 litre/2¼ pt/5½ cup bowl and heat, uncovered, on Full for 5 minutes, whisking every minute, until hot and smooth.

Piquant Sauce with Pickled Walnuts

Serves 4–6

Prepare as for Piquant Brown Sauce, but substitute 15 ml/1 tbsp chopped pickled walnuts for the capers.

Portuguese Sauce

Serves 6

The lovely flavour of this fresh tomato sauce does wondrous things to salmon and also cheers up roasted chicken and turkey.

30 ml/2 tbsp olive oil

1 onion, finely grated

2 rashers (slices) streaky bacon, finely chopped

1–2 garlic cloves, crushed

1 small carrot, grated

30 ml/2 tbsp plain (all-purpose) flour

5 tomatoes, blanched, skinned and chopped

45 ml/3 tbsp tomato purée (paste)

150 ml/¼ pt/2/3 cup boiling meat or vegetable stock

10 ml/2 tsp pickling spice, tied in a piece of muslin

10 ml/2 tsp dark soft brown sugar

5 ml/1 tsp salt

5 cm/2 in strip lemon peel

10 ml/2 tsp fresh lemon juice

Freshly ground black pepper

Put the oil, onion, bacon, garlic and carrot in a 2 litre/3½ pt/8½ cup bowl. Cook, uncovered, on Full for 4 minutes, stirring twice. Mix in the flour and cook on Full for 1 minute. Stir in all the remaining ingredients, adding pepper to taste. Cover with clingfilm (plastic wrap) and slit it twice to allow steam to escape. Cook on full for 7 minutes, turning twice. Allow to stand for 3 minutes. Strain into a clean dish. Cover with a plate and reheat on Full for 2–3 minutes before serving.

Rustic Tomato Sauce

Serves 4–6

30 ml/2 tbsp olive oil

1 onion, very finely chopped

2 celery stalks, finely chopped

1 rasher (slice) streaky bacon, finely chopped

1 small carrot, grated

1 garlic clove, crushed

25 ml/1½ tbsp plain (all-purpose) flour

400 g/14 oz/1 large can plum tomatoes, mashed

30 ml/2 tbsp tomato purée (paste)

10 ml/2 tsp dark soft brown sugar

1.5 ml/¼ tsp grated nutmeg

2.5 ml/½ tsp salt

150 ml/¼ pt/2/3 cup boiling stock or water

Put the oil in a 2 litre/3½ pt/8½ cup bowl. Mix in the onion, celery, bacon, carrot and garlic. Cook, uncovered, on Full for 4½ minutes, stirring twice. Mix in the flour. Cook, uncovered, on Full for 30 seconds. Add all the remaining ingredients and stir thoroughly to mix. Part-cover with a plate and cook on Full for 7 minutes, stirring three times. Allow to stand for 2 minutes.

Curried Turkey Sauce for Jacket Potatoes

Serves 6

15 ml/1 tbsp corn oil

2 onions, chopped

20 ml/4 tsp mild, medium or hot curry powder

350 g/12 oz/3 cups minced (ground) turkey

20 ml/4 tsp plain flour

150 ml/¼ pt/2/3 cup canned coconut milk

150 ml/¼ pt/2/3 cup water

30 ml/2 tbsp tomato purée (paste)

15 ml/1 tbsp fruit chutney

5 ml/1 tsp salt

Juice of 1 lime

30 ml/2 tbsp apple juice

150 ml/¼ pt/2/3 cup thick plain yoghurt

Pour the oil into a 1.25 litre/2¼ pt/5½ cup bowl. Heat on Full for 30 seconds. Mix in the onions and curry powder. Cook, uncovered, on Full for 5 minutes, stirring three times. Stir in the turkey. Cover with a plate and cook on Full for 6 minutes, stirring with a fork three or four times to keep the turkey crumbly. Mix in all the remaining ingredients except the yoghurt. Cover as before and cook on Full for 4 minutes, stirring twice. Allow to stand for 4 minutes. Spoon into split jacket potatoes and top each with a dollop of thick yoghurt.

Tandoori Turkey Sauce for Jacket Potatoes

Serves 6

Prepare as for Curried Turkey Sauce for Jacket Potatoes, but substitute tandoori powder for curry powder.

Hot Chilli Beef Sauce for Jacket Potatoes

Serves 6

60 ml/4 tbsp corn or sunflower oil

2 onions, chopped

2 cloves garlic, crushed

350 g/12 oz/3 cups lean minced (ground) beef

30 ml/2 tbsp plain (all-purpose) flour

2.5–10 ml/½–2 tsp chilli powder

30 ml/2 tbsp tomato purée (paste)

300 ml/½ pt/1¼ cups hot water

5 ml/1 tsp salt

45 ml/3 tbsp dry cider

Pour the oil into a 1.25 litre/2¼ pt/5½ cup dish. Mix in the onions and garlic. Cook, uncovered, on Full for 5 minutes, stirring twice. Stir in the beef. Cover with a plate and cook on Full for 6 minutes, stirring with a fork three or four times to keep the meat crumbly. Stir in the remaining ingredients. Cover with clingfilm (plastic wrap) and slit it twice to allow steam to escape. Cook on Full for 6 minutes, turning the dish twice, until bubbling. Allow to stand for 5 minutes. Stir round, then spoon into split jacket potatoes.

Chop House Sauce

Serves 4

An assertive sauce from Edwardian days for grilled chops, chicken and steaks. A little goes a long way, which is why the quantities are small.

15 ml/1 tbsp tomato ketchup (catsup)
5–10 ml/1–2 tsp anchovy essence (extract)
5 ml/1 tsp English made mustard
15 ml/1 tbsp wine vinegar
45 ml/3 tbsp double (heavy) cream
2.5 ml/½ tsp Worcestershire sauce
A dash of hot pepper sauce

Put all the ingredients in a 600 ml/1 pt/2½ cup measuring jug. Warm through, uncovered, on Full for 1¼ –1½ minutes, stirring twice, until hot but not boiling. Use straight away.

Hot Cheese and Carrot Sauce for Jacket Potatoes

Serves 4

A vegetarian sauce with a zippy temperament.

25 g/1 oz/2 tbsp butter or margarine

1 large carrot, grated

30 ml/2 tbsp plain (all-purpose) flour

300 ml/½ pt/1¼ cups warmed milk

5 ml/1 tsp mustard powder

1.5 ml/¼ tsp cayenne pepper

A pinch of ground nutmeg

2.5 ml/½ tsp salt

2.5 ml/½ tsp dried marjoram

50 g/2 oz/½ cup grated cheese

Put the butter or margarine in a 1.25 litre/2¼ pt/5½ cup dish. Melt, uncovered, on Defrost for 1 minute. Stir in the carrot. Cook, uncovered, on Full for 4 minutes, stirring twice. Mix in the flour. Cook, uncovered, on Full for 30 seconds, then gradually blend in the warmed milk. Cook, uncovered, on Full for 4 minutes, stirring vigorously every minute. Stir in the remaining ingredients. Cook on Full for 30 seconds. Stir round and spoon into split jacket potatoes.

Basting Sauces

Brushed over meat joints, poultry and foods on the barbecue, bastes increase browning and make them look more appetising. They also add to the flavour and can be used as a basis for gravy and savoury sauces.

Butter Baste

Makes about 60 ml/4 tbsp

25 g/1 oz/2 tbsp butter or margarine, at kitchen temperature
15 ml/1 tbsp tomato purée (paste)
5 ml/1 tsp paprika
5 ml/1 tsp Worcestershire sauce
5 ml/1 tsp light soft brown sugar

Melt the butter, uncovered, on Defrost for 1–1½ minutes. Stir in the remaining ingredients. Reheat on Defrost for 30 seconds and use as required.

Spicy Curry Baste

Makes about 60 ml/4 tbsp

Prepare as for Butter Baste, but stir in 5 ml/1 tsp mild curry powder, 5 ml/1 tsp mustard powder, 2.5 ml/½ tsp garlic salt and a pinch of turmeric with the remaining ingredients.

Jalapeno Mexican Barbecue Baste

Serves 6

You can't mistake the south-of-the-border kick from this one, which perks up barbecued pork and chicken like nothing else.

150 ml/¼ pt/2/3 cup French dressing

45 ml/3 tbsp tomato ketchup (catsup)

15 ml/1 tbsp soy sauce

15 ml/1 tbsp Worcestershire sauce

15 ml/1 tbsp jalapeno sauce

15 ml/1 tbsp fresh lime juice

2.5 ml/½ tsp dried mixed herbs

Put all the ingredients in a 600 ml/1 pt/2½ cup dish. Cover with a saucer and heat on Full for 2½ minutes. Stir round and use for basting.

Tomato Baste

Makes about 60 ml/4 tbsp

A non-fat baste, ideal for slimmers and those on low-fat diets and also with rich meats such as pork, duck and goose.

15 ml/1 tbsp tomato purée (paste)

5 ml/1 tsp English made mustard

5 ml/1 tsp malt vinegar

5 ml/1 tsp Worcestershire sauce

Thoroughly mix together all the ingredients in a jug and heat, uncovered, on Full for 10 seconds.

Dutch Butter Blender Cream

Serves 4–6

Lush to eat and a cream that can be made when you run out of fresh or fancy something a bit different. It can be whipped to peaks like whipping cream and melts over hot food like ice cream.

150 ml/¼ pt/2/3 cup full-cream milk
150 g/5 oz/2/3 cup Dutch unsalted (sweet) butter

Pour the milk into a bowl. Cut in the pieces of butter. Heat, uncovered on Full for 2½ minutes. Transfer carefully to a blender and run the machine for 1 minute. Return to the washed and dried bowl, cover and chill for 2–3 hours. Spoon over puddings or whip softly, if preferred.

Dutch Butter Blender Cream with Vanilla

Serves 4–6

Prepare as for Dutch Butter Blender Cream, but add 5 ml/1 tsp vanilla essence (extract) to the milk and butter in the blender.

Hot Chocolate Sauce

Serves 6

An old classic for ice cream, ice cream sundaes and profiteroles.

25 g/1 oz/2 tbsp butter

30 ml/2 tbsp light soft brown sugar

30 ml/2 tbsp cocoa (unsweetened chocolate) powder

30 ml/2 tbsp golden (light corn) syrup

30 ml/2 tbsp single (light) cream

5 ml/1 tsp vanilla essence (extract)

Put the butter in a 600 ml/1 pt/2½ cup dish. Melt, uncovered, on Full for 1 minute. Thoroughly stir in all the remaining ingredients. Cook, uncovered, on Defrost for 5 minutes, stirring every minute, until the sauce is smooth and hot.

Mocha Sauce

Serves 6

Prepare as for Hot Chocolate Sauce, but add 20 ml/4 tsp instant coffee powder or granules before heating.

Hot Chocolate and Orange Sauce

Serves 6

Prepare as for Hot Chocolate Sauce, but stir in 10 ml/2 tsp finely grated orange peel after cooking.

Hot Chocolate Peppermint Sauce

Serves 6

Prepare as for Hot Chocolate sauce, but add a few drops of peppermint essence (extract) after cooking.

Raspberry Coulis

Serves 6–8

A clear – almost glassy – brilliant red sauce beloved by chefs for its stunning effect.

350 g/12 oz/3 cups fresh raspberries
45 ml/3 tbsp caster (superfine) sugar
15 ml/1 tbsp cornflour (cornstarch)
75 ml/5 tbsp cold water
5 ml/1 tsp vanilla essence (extract)
5 ml/1 tsp lemon juice

Carefully rinse the raspberries, then put in a food processor or blender and work to a purée. Strain through fine-mesh sieve (strainer) to remove the seeds. Transfer to a 900 ml/1½ pt/3¾ cup bowl with the sugar. Mix the cornflour smoothly with the water. Add to the purée in the bowl. Cook, uncovered, on Full for 2½–3½ minutes, whisking every 30 seconds, until the mixture has thickened and is clear and bubbling gently. Stir in the vanilla and lemon juice and use cold.

Summer Fruit Coulis

Serves 6–8

Prepare as for Raspberry Coulis, but substitute a mixture of summer fruits for the raspberries.

Apricot Coulis

Serves 6–8

450 g/1 lb stoned (pitted) apricots

200 ml/7 fl oz/scant 1 cup cold water

60–75 ml/4–5 tbsp caster (superfine) sugar

15 ml/1 tbsp cornflour (cornstarch)

5 ml/1 tsp vanilla essence (extract)

5 ml/1 tsp lemon juice

Place the apricots in a dish with 60 ml/4 tbsp of the water. Cover with clingfilm (plastic wrap) and slit it twice to allow steam to escape. Cook on Full for 8–9 minutes until the fruit is tender. Transfer to a food processor or blender and work to a purée with another 60 ml/4 tbsp of the water. Transfer to a 900 ml/1½ pt/3¾ cup bowl with the sugar. Mix the cornflour smoothly with the remaining water. Add to the purée in the bowl. Cook, uncovered, on Full for 2½–3½ minutes, whisking every 30 seconds, until the mixture has thickened and is clear and bubbling gently. Stir in the vanilla and lemon juice and use cold.

Home-made Caramel Sauce

Serves 4

50 g/2 oz/¼ cup dark soft brown sugar

30 ml/2 tbsp cold water

15 ml/1 tbsp boiling water

Put the sugar and cold water into a measuring jug or bowl. Cook, uncovered, on Full for 2 minutes until boiling, watching carefully in case it starts to burn. Remove from the microwave and stir in the boiling water. Use hot as an ice cream topping or for Crème Caramel.

Egg Custard Sauce

Serves 4–6

A golden, glowing sauce, bliss over sweets like Summer Fruit Mould, steamed puddings, stewed fruits, even trifle.

600 ml/1 pt/2½ cups full-cream milk or half milk and half single (light) cream

10 ml/2 tsp cornflour (cornstarch)

15 ml/1 tbsp cold water

4 large eggs

45 ml/3 tbsp caster (superfine) sugar

5 ml/1 tsp vanilla essence (extract)

Pour the milk into a 1.25 litre/2¼ pt/5½ cup measuring jug and heat, uncovered, on Full for 2 minutes. Place the flour in a 1.25 litre/2¼ pt/5½ cup bowl and mix smoothly with the water. Break in the eggs, then add the sugar. Whisk until smooth, then gradually blend in the hot milk. Cook, uncovered, on Full for 5–5½ minutes, whisking every minute, until the sauce clings to the spatula or wooden spoon used for whisking. Mix in the vanilla essence.

Flavoured Egg Custard Sauce

Serves 4–6

Prepare as for Egg Custard Sauce, but substitute rum, sherry, almond or rose essence (extract) for the vanilla essence.

Lemon or Orange Custard

Serves 4–6

Prepare as for Egg Custard Sauce, but substitute 10 ml/2 tsp finely grated orange or lemon peel for the vanilla essence.

Brandy Sauce

Serves 4

Traditionally served on Christmas Pudding, also for mince pies.

25 g/1 oz/2 tbsp butter or margarine

30 ml/2 tbsp plain (all-purpose) flour

300 ml/½ pt/1¼ cups warmed milk

25–30 ml/1½–2 tbsp caster (superfine) sugar

25–30 ml/1½–2 tbsp brandy

Put the butter or margarine in a 900 ml/1½ pt/3¾ cup bowl. Melt, uncovered, on Defrost for 30–45 seconds. Stir in the flour. Cook on Full for 30 seconds. Gradually blend in the milk. Cook, uncovered, on Full for 4–5 minutes, beating every minute, until thickened and smooth. Mix in the sugar and cook, uncovered, on Full for 30 seconds. Stir in the brandy and serve.

Rum Sauce

Serves 4

Prepare as for Brandy Sauce, but substitute rum for the brandy.

Orange Sauce

Serves 4

An elusively scented sauce for any kind of light steamed pudding.

Prepare as for Brandy Sauce, but add 5 ml/1 tsp finely grated orange rind with the flour and substitute 15 ml/1 tbsp orange flower water for the brandy.

Sticky Toffee Sauce

Serves 4

Setting chewily on impact with ice cream, this is a heavenly sauce for any kind of sundae.

50 g/2 oz/¼ cup butter
40 g/1½ oz light soft brown sugar
50 g/2 oz marshmallows
15 ml/1 tbsp milk

Put all the ingredients in a 1.75 litre/3 pt/7½ cup bowl (the large size is necessary because the mixture rises as it cooks). Melt, uncovered, on Defrost for 2 minutes. Stir thoroughly. Heat on Full for a further 2½ minutes, stirring carefully three times. Use straight away as this sauce sets quickly.

Fresh Raspberry Sauce

Serves 4

Fresh and fragrant, a superior summer sauce for sundaes based on nectarines or peaches and vanilla ice cream.

10 ml/2 tsp cornflour (cornstarch)
150 ml/¼ pt/2/3 cup single (light) cream
30 ml/2 tbsp caster (superfine) sugar
225 g/8 oz/2 cups fresh raspberries, carefully rinsed
15 ml/1 tbsp cherry brandy

Put the cornflour in a 1.5 litre/2½ pt/6 cup bowl and mix smoothly with some of the cream. Stir in the remaining cream with the sugar and half the raspberries. Cook, uncovered, on Full for 4 minutes, stirring every minute. Fold in the remaining raspberries with the cherry brandy. Serve warm.

Chocolate Honey Raisin Sauce

Serves 6–8

Wonderful over coffee ice cream or orange sorbet.

50 g/2 oz/1/3 cup raisins

15 ml/1 tbsp boiling water

100 g/3½ oz plain (semi-sweet) chocolate

25 g/1 oz/2 tbsp butter

30 ml/2 tbsp single (light) cream

30 ml/2 tbsp thick honey

5 ml/1 tsp vanilla essence (extract)

Soak the raisins in the boiling water. Break up the chocolate and place in a small bowl with the butter. Melt, uncovered, on Defrost for about 3½ minutes. Stir in the cream, honey and vanilla. Heat, uncovered, on Full for 30–40 seconds. Drain the raisins and stir in.

Paella

Serves 6

1 kg/2¼ lb boned chicken breast

30 ml/2 tbsp olive oil

2 onions, chopped

2 garlic cloves, crushed

1 green (bell) pepper, seeded and chopped

225 g/8 oz/1 cup risotto rice

1 packet saffron powder or 5 ml/1 tsp turmeric

175 g/6 oz/1½ cups frozen peas

4 tomatoes, blanched and skinned

225 g/8 oz cooked mussels

75 g/3 oz/¾ cup cooked ham, cubed

125 g/4 oz/1 cup peeled prawns (shrimp)

600 ml/1 pt/2½ cups boiling water

7.5–10 ml/1½–2 tsp salt

Extra cooked mussels, cooked prawns and lemon wedges for garnishing

Arrange the chicken around the edge of a 25 cm/10 in diameter casserole dish (Dutch oven), leaving a hole in the centre. Cover with clingfilm (plastic wrap) and slit it twice to allow steam to escape. Cook on Full for 15 minutes. Drain off the liquid and reserve. Cube the chicken. Wash and dry the dish. Pour the oil into the dish and heat on Full for 1 minute. Stir in the onions, garlic and green pepper. Cook, uncovered, on Full for 4 minutes. Add all the remaining ingredients with the chicken and reserved liquor, stirring in well. Cover as before and cook on Full for 20 minutes, turning the dish three times. Allow to stand inside the oven for 10 minutes, then cook for a further 5 minutes. Uncover and garnish with mussels, prawns and lemon wedges.

Paella with Pimientos

Serves 6

Prepare as for Paella, but omit the mussels, and other seafood if preferred, and garnish with lemon slices, 200 g/7 oz drained canned pimientos, cut into strips, and extra peas.

Chicken Amandine

Serves 4

A typically North American short-cut recipe.

4 poussins (chickens), about 450 g/1 lb each

300 ml/10 fl oz/1 can condensed cream of mushroom soup

150 ml/¼ pt/2/3 cup medium-dry sherry

1 garlic clove, crushed

90 ml/6 tbsp toasted flaked (slivered) almonds

175 g/6 oz/¾ cup brown rice, boiled

Broccoli

Put the poussins, breast sides down and in a single layer, in a large, deep dish that will fit into the microwave. Cover with clingfilm (plastic wrap) and slit it twice to allow steam to escape. Cook on Full for 25 minutes, turning the dish four times. Turn the chickens over so that they are now breast sides up. Gently whisk the soup with the sherry and any chicken cooking juices. Mix in the garlic. Pour back over the chickens. Cover as before and cook on Full for 15 minutes, turning the dish three times. Allow to stand for 5 minutes. Transfer the chickens to warmed dinner plates and coat with the sauce. Sprinkle with the almonds and serve with the rice and broccoli.

Chicken Amandine with Tomato and Basil

Serves 4

Prepare as for Chicken Amandine, but substitute condensed cream of tomato soup for mushroom and marsala for the sherry. Add 6 torn basil leaves towards the end of the cooking time.

Chicken Divan

Serves 4

Another easy North American speciality, traditionally made with broccoli.

1 large head of broccoli, cooked

25 g/1 oz/2 tbsp butter or margarine

45 ml/3 tbsp plain (all-purpose) flour

150 ml/¼ pt/2/3 cup warm chicken stock

150 ml/¼ pt/2/3 cup single (light) cream

50 g/2 oz/½ cup Red Leicester cheese, grated

30 ml/2 tbsp dry white wine

5 ml/1 tsp mild made mustard

225 g/8 oz/2 cups cooked chicken, cubed

Salt

Ground nutmeg

45 ml/3 tbsp grated Parmesan cheese

Paprika

Separate the broccoli into florets and arrange over the base of a lightly buttered deep 25 cm/10 in diameter dish. In a separate dish, heat the butter or margarine on Full for 45–60 seconds until it sizzles. Stir in the flour and gradually blend in the warm stock and cream. Cook on Full for 4–5 minutes until bubbly and thickened, whisking every minute. Stir in the Red Leicester, wine, mustard and chicken. Add salt and nutmeg to taste. Spoon the sauce over the broccoli. Sprinkle with

Parmesan cheese and paprika. Cover with clingfilm (plastic wrap) and slit it twice to allow steam to escape. Reheat on Defrost for 8–10 minutes until piping hot.

Chicken in Cream Sauce with Celery

Serves 4

Prepare as for Chicken Divan, but substitute 400 g/14 oz/1 large can celery hearts, drained, for the broccoli. (The liquid from the can may be reserved for other recipes.)

Chicken in Cream Sauce with Crisps

Serves 4

Prepare as for Chicken Divan, but omit the cheese and paprika topping. Instead, sprinkle with 1 small bag of potato crisps (chips), coarsely crushed.

Chicken à la King

Serves 4

Another import from the USA and an innovative means of using leftover chicken.

40 g/1½ oz/3 tbsp butter or margarine
40 g/1½ oz/1½ tbsp plain (all-purpose) flour
300 ml/½ pt/1¼ cups warm chicken stock
60 ml/4 tbsp double (heavy) cream
1 canned red pimiento, cut into narrow strips
200 g/7 oz/scant 1 cup canned sliced mushrooms, drained
Salt and freshly ground black pepper
350 g/12 oz/2 cups cooked chicken, diced
15 ml/1 tbsp medium-dry sherry
Freshly made toast, to serve

Put the butter or margarine in a 1.5 litre/2½ pt/6 cup casserole dish (Dutch oven). Heat, uncovered, on Defrost for 1 minute. Stir in the flour, then gradually blend in the stock and cream. Cook, uncovered, on Full for 5–6 minutes until bubbling and thickened, whisking every minute. Stir in all the remaining ingredients and mix well. Cover with a plate and reheat on Full for 3 minutes. Allow to stand for 3 minutes before serving on toast.

Turkey à la King

Serves 4

Prepare as for Chicken à la King (above), but substitute cooked turkey for the chicken.

Chicken à la King with Cheese

Serves 4

Prepare as for Chicken à la King (above), but after reheating for 3 minutes, cover with 125 g/4 oz/1 cup grated Red Leicester cheese. Reheat, uncovered, on Full for a further 1–1½ minutes until the cheese melts.

Chicken à la King Shortcakes

Serves 4

Prepare as for Chicken à la King. Before serving, split open 4 large plain or cheese scones (biscuits) and put the bases on four warmed plates. Cover with the chicken mixture and top with the lids. Eat hot.

Slimmers' Chicken Liver Braise

Serves 4

A low-fat, low-starch main course that can be eaten with broccoli or cauliflower instead of potatoes.

15 ml/1 tbsp olive or sunflower oil

1 red (bell) pepper, seeded and thinly sliced

1 large carrot, thinly sliced

1 large onion, thinly sliced

2 large celery stalks, diagonally cut into thin slices

450 g/1 lb chicken livers, cut into bite-sized pieces

10 ml/2 tsp cornflour (cornstarch)

4 large tomatoes, blanched, skinned and coarsely chopped

Salt and freshly ground black pepper

Put the oil in a 1.75 litre/3 pt/7½ cup casserole dish (Dutch oven). Stir in the prepared vegetables and cook, uncovered, on Full for 5 minutes, stirring twice. Mix the liver into the vegetables and cook, uncovered, on Full for 3 minutes, stirring once. Stir in the cornflour, tomatoes and seasoning to taste. Cover with clingfilm (plastic wrap) and slit it twice to allow steam to escape. Cook on Full for 6 minutes, turning once.

Slimmers' Turkey Liver Braise

Serves 4

Prepare as for Slimmers' Chicken Liver Braise, but substitute turkey livers for the chicken livers.

Chicken Tetrazzini

Serves 4

175 g/6 oz/1½ cup short-cut macaroni

300 ml/10 fl oz/1 can condensed cream of chicken or mushroom soup

150 ml/¼ pt/2/3 cup milk

225 g/8 oz mushrooms, sliced

350 g/12 oz/2 cups cold cooked chicken, diced

15 ml/1 tbsp lemon juice

50 g/2 oz/¾ cup flaked (slivered) almonds

1.5 ml/¼ tsp ground nutmeg

75 g/3 oz/¾ cup Cheddar cheese, finely grated

Cook the macaroni as directed on the packet. Drain. Tip the soup into a buttered 1.75 litre/3 pt/7½ cup dish. Whisk in the milk. Heat, uncovered, on Full for 5–6 minutes until hot and bubbling lightly. Stir in the macaroni and all the remaining ingredients except the cheese. Cover with clingfilm (plastic wrap) and slit it twice to allow steam to escape. Cook on Full for 12 minutes, turning the dish three times. Uncover and sprinkle with the cheese. Brown conventionally under a hot grill (broiler).

Chicken and Mixed Vegetable Layer Casserole

Serves 4

4 large cooked potatoes, thinly sliced

3 cooked carrots, thinly sliced

125 g/4 oz/1 cup cooked peas

125 g/4 oz/1 cup cooked sweetcorn

4 portions chicken, 225 g/8 oz each, skinned

300 ml/10 fl oz/1 can condensed cream of celery soup, or other flavour to taste

45 ml/3 tbsp medium-dry sherry

30 ml/2 tbsp single (light) cream

1.5 ml/¼ tsp grated nutmeg

75 g/3 oz/1¼ cups cornflakes, coarsely crushed

Cover the base of a buttered deep 25 cm/10 in diameter dish with the potato and carrot slices. Sprinkle with the peas and sweetcorn and top with the chicken. Cover with clingfilm (plastic wrap) and slit it twice to allow steam to escape. Cook on Full for 8 minutes, turning the dish four times. Whisk the soup with all the remaining ingredients except the cornflakes. Spoon over the chicken. Cover as before and cook on Full for 11 minutes, turning the dish twice. Allow to stand for 5 minutes. Uncover and sprinkle with the cornflakes before serving.

Honey Chicken on Rice

Serves 4

25 g/1 oz/2 tbsp butter or margarine

1 large onion, chopped

6 streaky bacon rashers (slices), chopped

75 g/3 oz/1/3 cup easy-cook long-grain rice

300 ml/½ pt/1¼ cups hot chicken stock

Freshly ground black pepper

4 boned chicken breasts, 175 g/6 oz each

Finely grated peel and juice of 1 orange

30 ml/2 tbsp dark clear honey

5 ml/1 tsp paprika

5 ml/1 tsp Worcestershire sauce

Put the butter or margarine in a deep 20 cm/8 in diameter dish. Heat, uncovered, on Full for 1 minute. Stir in the onion, bacon, rice, stock and pepper to taste. Arrange the chicken in a ring on top. Beat together the orange peel and juice, honey, paprika and Worcestershire sauce. Spoon half over the chicken. Cover with clingfilm (plastic wrap) and slit it twice to allow steam to escape. Cook on Full for 9 minutes, turning the dish three times. Uncover. Baste the chicken with the remaining honey mixture. Cook, uncovered, on Full for 5 minutes. Allow to stand for 3 minutes before serving.

Chicken in White Rum Sauce with Lime

Serves 4

25 g/1 oz/2 tbsp butter or margarine

10 ml/2 tsp corn or sunflower oil

1 leek, very thinly sliced

1 garlic clove, crushed

75 g/3 oz/¾ cup lean ham, chopped

675 g/1½ lb boned chicken breast, cut into bite-sized pieces

3 tomatoes, blanched, skinned and coarsely chopped

30 ml/2 tbsp white rum

5 cm/2 in strip lime peel

Juice of 1 sweet orange

Salt

150 ml/¼ pt/2/3 cup plain yoghurt

Watercress (optional)

Put the butter or margarine and oil in a 23 cm/9 in diameter casserole dish (Dutch oven). Heat, uncovered, on Full for 1 minute. Stir in the leek, garlic and ham. Cook, uncovered, on Full for 4 minutes, stirring twice. Mix in the chicken. Cover with a plate and cook on Full for 7 minutes, turning the dish twice. Add all remaining ingredients except the yoghurt and watercress, if using. Cover with clingfilm (plastic wrap) and slit it twice to allow steam to escape. Cook on Full for 8 minutes, turning the dish four times. Uncover. Combine the yoghurt with some of the liquid from the dish until smooth and creamy, then pour over the chicken. Reheat, uncovered, on Full for 1½ minutes. Discard the lime peel. Serve garnished with watercress, if liked.

Chicken in Brandy Sauce with Orange

Serves 4

Prepare as for Chicken in White Rum Sauce with Lime, but substitute brandy for the rum and orange peel for the lime. Use 60 ml/4 tbsp ginger ale instead of the orange juice.

Drumsticks in Barbecue Sauce with Baby Pasta

Serves 4

900 g/2 lb chicken drumsticks

2 onions, chopped

2 celery stalks, chopped

30 ml/2 tbsp wholegrain mustard

2.5 ml/½ tsp paprika

5 ml/1 tsp Worcestershire sauce

400 g/14 oz/1 large can chopped tomatoes in tomato juice

125 g/4 oz/1 cup any small pasta

7.5 ml/1½ tsp salt

Arrange the drumsticks, like the spokes of a wheel, in a deep 25 cm/10 in diameter dish, with the bony ends towards the centre. Cover with clingfilm (plastic wrap) and slit it twice to allow steam to escape. Cook on Full for 8 minutes, turning the dish three times. Meanwhile, place the vegetables in a bowl and stir in the remaining ingredients. Remove the dish of chicken from the microwave, uncover and pour the chicken cooking juices into the vegetable mixture. Mix well. Spoon over the drumsticks. Cover as before and cook on Full for 15 minutes, turning the dish three times. Allow to stand for 5 minutes before serving.

Chicken in Mexican Mole Sauce

Serves 4

4 boned chicken breasts, 175 g/6 oz each, skinned

30 ml/2 tbsp corn oil

1 large onion, finely chopped

1 green (bell) pepper, seeded and chopped

1 garlic clove, crushed

30 ml/2 tbsp plain (all-purpose) flour

3 whole cloves

1 bay leaf

2.5 ml/½ tsp ground cinnamon

5 ml/1 tsp salt

150 ml/¼ pt/2/3 cup tomato juice

50 g/2 oz/½ cup plain (semi-sweet) chocolate, broken into pieces

175 g/6 oz/¾ cup long-grain rice, boiled

15 ml/1 tbsp garlic butter

Arrange the chicken round the edge of a deep 20 cm/8 in diameter dish. Cover with clingfilm (plastic wrap) and slit it twice to allow steam to escape. Cook on Full for 6 minutes. Allow to stand while preparing the sauce. In a separate dish, heat the oil, uncovered, on Full for 1 minute. Stir in the onion, green pepper and garlic. Cook, uncovered, on Full for 3 minutes, stirring twice. Stir in the flour, then the cloves, bay leaf, cinnamon, salt and tomato juice. Cook, uncovered, on Full for 4 minutes, stirring every minute. Remove from the microwave. Add the chocolate and stir in thoroughly. Cook, uncovered, on Full for 30 seconds. Uncover the chicken and coat with the hot sauce. Cover as before and cook on Full for 8 minutes. Allow to stand for 5 minutes. Serve with the rice, forked with the garlic butter.

Chicken Wings in Barbecue Sauce with Baby Pasta

Serves 4

Prepare as for Drumsticks in Barbecue Sauce with Baby Pasta, but substitute chicken wings for the drumsticks.

Chicken Jambalaya

Serves 3–4

Hotfoot from Louisiana this is a stunning rice and chicken dish, a relative of paella.

2 boned chicken breasts
50 g/2 oz/¼ cup butter or margarine
2 large onions, chopped
1 red (bell) pepper, seeded and chopped
4 celery stalks, chopped
2 garlic cloves, crushed
225 g/8 oz/1 cup easy-cook long-grain rice
400 g/14 oz/1 large can chopped tomatoes in tomato juice
10–15 ml/2–3 tsp salt

Arrange the chicken round the edge of a deep 25 cm/10 in diameter dish. Cover with clingfilm (plastic wrap) and slit it twice to allow steam to escape. Cook on Full for 7 minutes. Allow to stand for 2 minutes. Transfer the chicken to a board and cut into cubes. Pour the chicken cooking juices into a jug and reserve. Wash and dry the dish, add the butter and melt, uncovered, on Full for 1½ minutes. Stir in the reserved liquid, the chicken, prepared vegetables, garlic, rice and tomatoes. Season to taste with the salt. Cover as before and cook on Full for 20–25 minutes until the rice grains are dry and have absorbed all the moisture. Allow to stand for 5 minutes, fluff up with a fork and serve straight away.

Turkey Jambalaya

Serves 3–4

Prepare as for Chicken Jambalaya, but substitute turkey breast for chicken.

Chicken with Chestnuts

Serves 4

25 g/1 oz/2 tbsp butter or margarine

2 large onions, peeled and grated

430 g/15 oz/1 large can unsweetened chestnut purée

2.5 ml/½ tsp salt

4 skinned and boned chicken breasts, 175 g/6 oz each

3 tomatoes, blanched, skinned and sliced

30 ml/2 tbsp chopped parsley

Red cabbage and boiled potatoes, to serve

Put the butter or margarine in a deep 20 cm/8 in diameter dish. Melt, uncovered, on Defrost for 1½ minutes. Mix in the onions. Cook, uncovered, on Full for 4 minutes. Spoon in the chestnut purée and salt and mix smoothly, blending well with the onions. Spread in an even layer over the base of the dish and arrange the chicken breasts on top round the edge of the dish. Top with tomato slices and sprinkle with the parsley. Cover with clingfilm (plastic wrap) and slit it twice to allow steam to escape. Cook on Full for 15 minutes, turning the dish three times. Allow to stand for 4 minutes. Serve with red cabbage and potatoes.

Chicken Gumbo

Serves 6

A cross between a soup and a stew, the Gumbo is Southern comfort and one of Louisiana's best exports. Its basis is okra (ladies' fingers) and a brown roux, with the addition of vegetables, spices, stock and chicken.

50 g/2 oz/¼ cup butter

50 g/2 oz/½ cup plain (all-purpose) flour

900 ml/1½ pts/3¾ cups hot chicken stock

350 g/12 oz okra (ladies' fingers), topped and tailed

2 large onions, finely chopped

2 garlic cloves, crushed

2 large celery stalks, thinly sliced

1 green (bell) pepper, seeded and chopped

15–20 ml/3–4 tsp salt

10 ml/2 tsp ground coriander (cilantro)

5 ml/1 tsp turmeric

5–10 ml/1–2 tsp ground allspice

30 ml/2 tbsp lemon juice

2 bay leaves

5–10 ml/1–2 tsp hot pepper sauce

450 g/1 lb/4 cups cooked chicken, chopped

175 g/6 oz/¾ cups long-grain rice, boiled

Put the butter in a 2.5 litre/4½ pt/11 cup casserole dish (Dutch oven). Heat, uncovered, on Full for 2 minutes. Stir in the flour. Cook, uncovered, on Full for 7 minutes, stirring every minute, until the mixture is a light brown roux, the colour of a well-baked biscuit (cookie). Gradually blend in the hot stock. Slice each okra into eight pieces and add to the casserole with all the remaining ingredients except the chicken and rice. Cover with clingfilm (plastic wrap) and slit it twice to allow steam to escape. Cook on Full for 15 minutes. Stir in the chicken. Cover as before and cook on Full for 15 minutes. Allow to stand for 5 minutes. Stir round and ladle into soup bowls. Add a mound of rice to each.

Turkey Gumbo

Serves 6

Prepare as for Chicken Gumbo, but substitute cooked turkey for the chicken.

Chicken Breasts with Brown Orange Baste

Serves 4

60 ml/4 tbsp orange jam (conserve) or fine-cut marmalade

15 ml/1 tbsp malt vinegar

15 ml/1 tbsp soy sauce

1 garlic clove, crushed

2.5 ml/½ tsp ground ginger

7.5 ml/1½ tsp cornflour (cornstarch)

4 boned chicken breasts, 200 g/7 oz each, skinned

Chinese noodles, boiled

Combine all the ingredients except the chicken and noodles in a small dish. Heat, uncovered, on Full for 50 seconds. Arrange the chicken breasts round the edge of a deep 20 cm/8 in diameter dish. Spoon over half the baste. Cover with a plate and cook on Full for 8 minutes, turning the dish twice. Turn the breasts over and brush with the remaining baste. Cover as before and cook on Full for a further 8 minutes. Allow to stand for 4 minutes, then serve with Chinese noodles.

Chicken in Creamy Pepper Sauce

Serves 6

25 g/1 oz/2 tbsp butter or margarine

1 small onion, finely chopped

4 boned chicken breasts

15 ml/1 tbsp cornflour (cornstarch)

30 ml/2 tbsp cold water

15 ml/1 tbsp tomato purée (paste)

20–30 ml/4–6 tsp bottled or canned Madagascan green peppercorns

150 ml/¼ pt/2/3 cup soured (dairy sour) cream

5 ml/1 tsp salt

275 g/10 oz/1¼ cup long-grain rice, boiled

Put the butter or margarine in a deep 20 cm/8 in diameter dish. Melt, uncovered, on Full for 45–60 seconds. Add the onion. Cook, uncovered, on Full for 2 minutes. Cut the chicken breasts across the grain into 2.5 cm/1 in wide strips. Mix well into the butter and onions. Cover with clingfilm (plastic wrap) and slit it twice to allow steam to escape. Cook on Full for 6 minutes, turning the dish three times. Meanwhile, mix the cornflour smoothly with the cold water. Stir in all the remaining ingredients except the rice. Combine with the chicken and onion, moving the mixture to the edges of the dish and leaving a small hollow in the centre. Cover as before and cook on Full for 8 minutes, turning the dish four times. Allow to stand for 4 minutes. Stir round before serving with the rice.

Turkey in Creamy Pepper Sauce

Serves 6

Prepare as for Chicken in Creamy Pepper Sauce, but substitute turkey breast for the chicken.

Woodland Chicken

Serves 4

4 skinned chicken quarters, 225 g/8 oz each

30 ml/2 tbsp corn or sunflower oil

175 g/6 oz streaky bacon rashers (slices), chopped

1 onion, chopped

175 g/6 oz button mushrooms, sliced

300 ml/½ pt/1¼ cups sieved tomatoes (passata)

15 ml/1 tbsp brown vinegar

15 ml/1 tbsp lemon juice

30 ml/2 tbsp light soft brown sugar

5 ml/1 tsp prepared mustard

30 ml/2 tbsp Worcestershire sauce

Chopped coriander (cilantro) leaves, to garnish

Arrange the chicken round the edge of a 25 cm/10 in diameter casserole dish (Dutch oven). Cover with clingfilm (plastic wrap) and slit it twice to allow steam to escape. Pour the oil into a separate dish and heat, uncovered, on Full for 1 minute. Add the bacon, onion and mushrooms. Cook, uncovered, on Full for 5 minutes. Mix in all the remaining ingredients. Cook the covered chicken on Full for 9 minutes, turning the dish twice. Uncover and coat with the vegetable mixture. Cover as before and cook on Full for 10 minutes, turning the dish three times. Allow to stand for 5 minutes. Sprinkle with coriander before serving.

Chicken with Apples and Raisins

Serves 4

25 g/1 oz/2 tbsp butter or margarine

900 g/2 lb chicken joints

2 onions, chopped

3 Cox's apples, peeled and chopped

30 ml/2 tbsp raisins

1 garlic clove, chopped

30 ml/2 tbsp plain (all-purpose) flour

250 ml/8 fl oz/1 cup shandy

2 beef stock cubes

2.5 ml/½ tsp dried thyme

Salt and freshly ground black pepper

30 ml/2 tbsp chopped parsley

Put the butter or margarine in a 25 cm/10 in diameter casserole dish (Dutch oven). Melt, uncovered, on Defrost for 1–1½ minutes. Add the chicken. Cover with clingfilm (plastic wrap) and slit it twice to allow steam to escape. Cook on Full for 8 minutes. Uncover and turn the chicken over. Cover as before and cook on Full for a further 7 minutes. Uncover and sprinkle with the onions, apples, raisins and garlic. Blend the flour smoothly with some of the shandy, then mix in the remaining shandy. Crumble in the gravy cubes, add the thyme and season to taste. Pour over the chicken. Cover as before and cook on Full for 8 minutes until the liquid bubbles and has thickened slightly. Allow to stand for 5 minutes. Uncover and sprinkle with the parsley.

Chicken with Pears and Raisins

Serves 4

Prepare as for Chicken with Apples and Raisins, but substitute pears for the apples and cider for the shandy.

Grapefruit Chicken

Serves 4

2 celery stalks

30 ml/2 tbsp butter or margarine

1 large onion, finely grated

4 large chicken joints, 1 kg/2¼ lb in all, skinned

Plain (all-purpose) flour

1 large pink grapefruit

150 ml/¼ pt/2/3 cup white or rosé wine

30 ml/2 tbsp tomato purée (paste)

1.5 ml/¼ tsp dried rosemary

5 ml/1 tsp salt

Cut the celery across the grain into narrow strips. Put the butter or margarine in a deep 25 cm/10 in diameter dish. Melt, uncovered, on Full for 30 seconds. Mix in the onion and celery. Cook, uncovered, on Full for 6 minutes. Dust the chicken lightly with flour, then arrange round the edge of the dish. Cover with clingfilm (plastic wrap) and slit it twice to allow steam to escape. Cook on Full for 10 minutes, turning the dish three times. Meanwhile, peel the grapefruit and separate into segments by cutting between the membranes. Uncover the chicken and scatter the grapefruit segments over. Beat the wine with the tomato purée, rosemary and salt and pour over the chicken. Cover as before and cook on Full for 10 minutes. Allow to stand for 5 minutes before serving.

Hungarian Chicken and Mixed Vegetables

Serves 4

25 g/1 oz/2 tbsp butter or lard

2 large onions, chopped

1 small green (bell) pepper

3 small courgettes (zucchini), thinly sliced

450 g/1 lb boned chicken breast, cubed

15 ml/1 tbsp paprika

45 ml/3 tbsp tomato purée (paste)

150 ml/¼ pt/2/3 cup soured (dairy sour) cream

5–7.5 ml/1–1½ tsp salt

Put the butter or lard in a 25 cm/10 in diameter casserole dish (Dutch oven). Heat, uncovered, on Defrost for 1–1½ minutes. Stir in the onions. Cook, uncovered, on Full for 3 minutes. Mix in the green pepper, courgettes, chicken, paprika and tomato purée. Cover with clingfilm (plastic wrap) and slit it twice to allow steam to escape. Cook on Full for 5 minutes, turning the dish three times. Uncover. Gradually work in the soured cream and salt. Cover as before and cook on Full for 8 minutes. Allow to stand for 5 minutes, then stir round and serve.

Chicken Bourguignonne

Serves 6

A gourmet main course, more traditionally made with beef but lighter with chicken.

25 g/1 oz/2 tbsp butter or margarine

2 onions, chopped

1 garlic clove, crushed

750 g/1½ lb chicken breast, cubed

30 ml/2 tbsp cornflour (cornstarch)

5 ml/1 tsp continental mustard

2.5 ml/½ tsp dried mixed herbs

300 ml/½ pt/1¼ cups burgundy wine

225 g/8 oz mushrooms, thinly sliced

5–7.5 ml/1–1½ tsp salt

45 ml/3 tbsp chopped parsley

Put the butter or margarine in a 25 cm/10 in diameter casserole dish (Dutch oven). Melt, uncovered, on Defrost for 1½ minutes. Mix in the onions and garlic. Cover with a plate and cook on Full for 3 minutes. Uncover and mix in the chicken. Cover with clingfilm (plastic wrap) and slit it twice to allow steam to escape. Cook on Full for 8 minutes. Mix the cornflour and mustard smoothly with some of the burgundy, then stir in the remainder. Pour over the chicken. Sprinkle with the mushrooms and salt. Cover as before and cook on Full for 8–9 minutes, turning the dish four times, until the sauce has thickened and is beginning to bubble. Allow to stand for 5 minutes, then stir round and sprinkle with the parsley before serving.

Chicken Fricassée

Serves 6

A revival of a twenties and thirties special-occasion chicken main course, always eaten with white rice fluffed with butter and grilled (broiled) bacon rolls. It needs a large microwave.

1.5 kg/3 lb chicken joints, skinned

1 onion, cut into 8 wedges

2 large celery stalks, thickly sliced

1 small carrot, thinly sliced

2 thick slices lemon

1 small bay leaf

2 whole cloves

Parsley sprigs

10 ml/2 tsp salt

300 ml/½ pt/1¼ cups hot water

150 ml/¼ pt/2/3 cup single (light) cream

40 g/1½ oz/3 tbsp butter or margarine

40 g/1½ oz/1½ tbsp plain (all-purpose) flour

Juice of 1 small lemon

Salt and freshly ground black pepper

Arrange the chicken in a 30 cm/12 in diameter casserole dish (Dutch oven). Add the onion, celery and carrot to the dish with the lemon slices, bay leaf, cloves and 1 parsley sprig. Sprinkle with the salt and add the water. Cover with clingfilm (plastic wrap) and slit it twice to allow steam to escape. Cook on Full for 24 minutes, turning the dish three times. Lift out the chicken. Remove the meat from the bones and cut into bite-sized pieces. Strain the liquid from the dish and reserve 300 ml/½ pt/1¼ cups. Mix in the cream. Place the butter in a large shallow dish. Melt, uncovered, on Full for 1½ minutes. Stir in the flour, then gradually blend in the warm stock and cream mixture. Cook, uncovered, on Full for 5–6 minutes, whisking every minute, until thickened and bubbling. Add the lemon juice, stir in the chicken and season to taste. Cover as before and reheat on Full for 5 minutes, turning the dish twice. Allow to stand for 4 minutes before garnishing with parsley sprigs and serving.

Chicken Fricassée with Wine

Serves 6

Prepare as for Chicken Fricassée, but use only 150 ml/¼ pt/2/3 cup reserved stock and add 150 ml/¼ pt/2/3 cup dry white wine.

Chicken Supreme

Serves 6

Prepare as for Chicken Fricassée. After reheating for 5 minutes at the end and then standing, beat in 2 egg yolks mixed with an extra 15 ml/1 tbsp cream. The heat from the mixture will cook the yolks.

Coq au Vin

Serves 6

50 g/2 oz/¼ cup butter or margarine

1.5 kg/3 lb chicken joints, skinned

1 large onion, finely chopped

1 garlic clove, crushed

30 ml/2 tbsp plain (all-purpose) flour

300 ml/½ pt/1¼ cups dry red wine

1 beef stock cube

5 ml/1 tsp salt

12 shallots or pickled onions

60 ml/4 tbsp chopped parsley

1.5 ml/¼ tsp dried thyme

Boiled potatoes and Brussels sprouts, to serve

Put the butter or margarine in a 30 cm/12 in diameter casserole dish (Dutch oven). Heat, uncovered, on Full for 1 minute. Add the chicken pieces and turn them over once so that all pieces are coated with butter but keep in a single layer. Cover with clingfilm (plastic wrap) and slit it twice to allow steam to escape. Cook on Full for 15 minutes, turning the dish three times. Uncover and sprinkle the chicken with the onion and garlic. Gradually mix the flour smoothly with the wine, whisking, if necessary, to remove lumps. Crumble in the stock cube and add the salt. Pour the wine mixture over the chicken. Surround with the shallots or onions and sprinkle with the parsley and thyme. Cover as before and cook on Full for 20 minutes, turning the dish three times. Allow to stand for 6 minutes. Eat with boiled potatoes and Brussels sprouts.

Coq au Vin with Mushrooms

Serves 6

Prepare as for Coq au Vin, but substitute 125 g/4 oz button mushrooms for the shallots or pickled onions.

Coq au Cola

Serves 6

Prepare as for Coq au Vin, but substitute cola for the wine to make the dish more suitable for children.

Drumsticks with Devilled Coating

Serves 4

15 ml/1 tbsp English mustard powder

10 ml/2 tsp hot curry powder

10 ml/2 tsp paprika

1.5 ml/¼ tsp hot cayenne pepper

2.5 ml/½ tsp salt

1 kg/2¼ lb chicken drumsticks (about 12)

45 ml/3 tbsp garlic butter

Mix together the mustard, curry powder, paprika, cayenne and salt. Use to coat all sides of the drumsticks. Arrange in a deep 25 cm/10 in diameter dish like the spokes of a wheel, with the bony ends towards the centre. Melt the butter, uncovered, on Full for 1 minute. Coat the drumsticks with the melted butter. Cover with clingfilm (plastic wrap) and slit it twice to allow steam to escape. Cook on Full for 16 minutes, turning the dish twice.

Chicken Cacciatore

Serves 6

An Italian dish, which translates to 'hunter's chicken'.

1.5 kg/3 lb chicken pieces

15 ml/1 tbsp olive oil

1 large onion, finely chopped

1 garlic clove, crushed

30 ml/2 tbsp plain (all-purpose) flour

5 tomatoes, blanched, skinned and chopped

150 ml/¼ pt/2/3 cup hot stock

45 ml/3 tbsp tomato purée (paste)

15 ml/1 tbsp brown table sauce

125 g/4 oz mushrooms, sliced

10 ml/2 tsp salt

10 ml/2 tsp dark soft brown sugar

45 ml/3 tbsp marsala or medium-dry sherry

Creamed potatoes and mixed salad, to serve

Place the chicken in a 30 cm/12 in diameter casserole dish (Dutch oven). Cover with clingfilm (plastic wrap) and slit it twice to allow steam to escape. Cook on Full for 15 minutes, turning the dish twice. Meanwhile, make the sauce conventionally. Pour the oil into a saucepan and add the onion and garlic. Fry (sauté) gently until lightly golden. Stir in the flour, then add the tomatoes, stock, purée and brown sauce. Cook, stirring, until the sauce comes to the boil and thickens.

Stir in all the remaining ingredients and pour over the chicken. Cover as before and cook on Full for 20 minutes, turning the dish three times. Allow to stand for 5 minutes. Serve with creamed potatoes and a mixed salad.

Chicken Chasseur

Serves 6

Prepare as for Chicken Cacciatore, but substitute dry white wine for the marsala or sherry.

Chicken Marengo

Serves 6

Invented in about 1800 by Napoleon Bonaparte's personal chef on the battlefields after the Austrian defeat at the Battle of Marengo, near Verona in northern Italy.

Prepare as for Chicken Cacciatore, but use only 50 g/2 oz mushrooms and substitute dry white wine for the marsala or sherry. When stirring in all the remaining ingredients, add 12–16 small stoned (pitted) black olives and 60 ml/4 tbsp chopped parsley.

Sesame Chicken

Serves 4

50 g/2 oz/¼ cup butter or margarine, softened

15 ml/1 tbsp mild mustard

5 ml/1 tsp garlic purée (paste)

5 ml/1 tsp tomato purée (paste)

90 ml/6 tbsp sesame seeds, lightly toasted

4 chicken portions, each 225 g/8 oz, skinned

Cream the butter or margarine with the mustard and the garlic and tomato purées. Stir in the sesame seeds. Spread the mixture evenly over the chicken. Arrange in a deep 25 cm/10 in diameter dish, leaving a hollow in the centre. Cook on Full for 16 minutes, turning the dish four times. Allow to stand for 5 minutes before serving.

Country Captain

Serves 6

An East Indian mild chicken curry, brought to the southern states of North America long ago by a much-travelled sea captain. It has become a kind of oriental standby in the USA.

50 g/2 oz/¼ cup butter or margarine

2 onions, chopped

1 celery stalk, chopped

1.5 kg/3 lb chicken joints, skinned

15 ml/1 tbsp plain (all-purpose) flour

15 ml/1 tbsp mild curry powder

60 ml/4 tbsp almonds, blanched, skinned, halved and lightly toasted

1 small green (bell) pepper, seeded and finely chopped

45 ml/3 tbsp sultanas (golden raisins)

10 ml/2 tsp salt

400 g/14 oz/1 large can chopped tomatoes

5 ml/1 tsp sugar

275 g/10 oz/1¼ cups long-grain rice, boiled

Put the butter or margarine in a 30 cm/12 in diameter casserole dish (Dutch oven). Heat, uncovered, on Full for 1½ minutes. Add the onions and celery and stir well. Cook, uncovered, on Full for 3 minutes, stirring twice. Add the chicken joints and toss in the butter and vegetable mixture until well coated. Sprinkle with the flour, curry powder, almonds, pepper and sultanas. Cover with clingfilm (plastic wrap) and slit it twice to allow steam to escape. Cook on Full for 8 minutes. Combine the salt with the tomatoes and sugar. Uncover the chicken and spoon the tomatoes over. Cover as before and cook on Full for 21 minutes, turning the dish twice. Allow to stand for 5 minutes before serving with the rice.

Serves 6

6 chicken joints, 225 g/8 oz each, skinned

Plain (all-purpose) flour

50 g/2 oz/¼ cup butter or margarine

3 rashers (slices) bacon, chopped

2 large onions, chopped

2 garlic cloves, crushed

15 ml/1 tbsp capers, chopped

400 g/14 oz/1 large can chopped tomatoes

15 ml/1 tbsp dark soft brown sugar

5 ml/1 tsp dried mixed herbs

15 ml/1 tbsp tomato purée (paste)

15 ml/1 tbsp chopped basil leaves

15 ml/1 tbsp chopped parsley

Dust the chicken joints with flour. Put the butter or margarine in a 30 cm/12 in diameter casserole dish (Dutch oven). Heat, uncovered, on Full for 2 minutes. Stir in the bacon, onions, cloves and capers. Cook, uncovered, on Full for 4 minutes, stirring twice. Add the chicken and toss until well coated with the butter or margarine mixture. Cover with clingfilm (plastic wrap) and slit it twice to allow steam to escape. Cook on Full for 12 minutes, turning the dish three times. Uncover and add the remaining ingredients, mixing in well. Cover as before and cook on Full for 18 minutes. Allow to stand for 6 minutes before serving.

Chicken Paprikas

Serves 4

Pronounced paprikash, this chicken fantasy is a relative of gulas or goulash, one of Hungary's most renowned dishes.

1.5 kg/3 lb chicken pieces

1 large onion, chopped

1 green (bell) pepper, seeded and chopped

1 garlic clove, crushed

30 ml/2 tbsp corn oil or melted lard

45 ml/3 tbsp plain (all-purpose) flour

15 ml/1 tbsp paprika

300 ml/½ pt/1¼ cups warm chicken stock

30 ml/2 tbsp tomato purée (paste)

5 ml/1 tsp dark soft brown sugar

2.5 ml/½ tsp caraway seeds

5 ml/1 tsp salt

150 ml/5 fl oz/2/3 cup crème fraîche

Small pasta shapes, boiled

Place the chicken pieces in a 30 cm/12 in diameter casserole dish (Dutch oven). Cover with clingfilm (plastic wrap) and slit it twice to allow steam to escape. Cook on Full for 15 minutes, turning the dish twice. Meanwhile, make the sauce conventionally. Put the onion, pepper, garlic and oil into a saucepan (skillet) and fry (sauté) gently until the vegetables are soft but not browned. Stir in the flour and paprika, then gradually blend in the stock. Bring to the boil, stirring. Stir in the remaining ingredients except the crème fraîche and pasta. Uncover the chicken and coat with the sauce, working in some of the juices already in the dish. Top with spoonfuls of crème fraîche. Cover as before and cook on Full for 20 minutes, turning the dish three times. Serve with small pasta.

Shades-of-the-East Chicken

Serves 6–8

Indian and Indonesian influences and tastes unite in this outstandingly grand chicken recipe.

15 ml/1 tbsp groundnut (peanut) oil

3 medium onions, chopped

2 garlic cloves, crushed

900 g/2 lb boned chicken breasts, skinned and cut into narrow strips

15 ml/1 tbsp cornflour (cornstarch)

60 ml/4 tbsp crunchy peanut butter

150 ml/¼ pt/2/3 cup water

7.5 ml/1½ tsp salt

10 ml/2 tsp mild curry paste

2.5 ml/½ tsp ground coriander (cilantro)

2.5 ml/½ tsp ground ginger

Seeds from 5 cardamom pods

60 ml/4 tbsp salted peanuts, coarsely-chopped

2 tomatoes, cut into wedges

Heat the oil in a 25 cm/10 in diameter casserole dish (Dutch oven), uncovered, on Full for 1 minute. Add the onions and garlic and cook, uncovered, on Full for 3 minutes, stirring twice. Mix in the chicken and cook, uncovered, on Full for 3 minutes, stirring with a fork every minute to separate. Sprinkle in the cornflour. Work in all the remaining ingredients except the peanuts and tomatoes. Cover with clingfilm (plastic wrap) and slit it twice to allow steam to escape. Cook on Full for 19 minutes, turning the dish four times. Allow to stand for 5 minutes. Stir round and garnish with the peanuts and tomato wedges before serving.

Nasi Goreng

Serves 6

A Dutch-Indonesian speciality.

175 g/6 oz/¾ cup easy-cook long-grain rice

50 g/2 oz/¼ cup butter or margarine

2 onions, chopped

2 leeks, white part only, very thinly sliced

1 green chilli, seeded and chopped (optional)

350 g/12 oz/3 cups cold cooked chicken, coarsely chopped

30 ml/2 tbsp soy sauce

1 Classic Omelette, cut into strips

1 large tomato, cut into wedges

Cook the rice as directed on the packet. Allow to cool. Put the butter or margarine in a 25 cm/10 in diameter casserole dish (Dutch oven). Heat, uncovered, on Full for 1 minute. Stir in the onions, leeks and chilli, if using. Cook, uncovered, on Full for 4 minutes. Stir in the rice, chicken and soy sauce. Cover with a plate and cook on Full for 6–7 minutes, stirring three times, until piping hot. Garnish with a criss-cross pattern of omelette strips and tomato wedges.

Roast Turkey

SERVES 6

1 turkey, size as required (allow 350 g/12 oz) uncooked weight per person)
Baste

Cover the wing tips and ends of the legs with foil. Stand the turkey, breast side down, in a dish large enough to hold the bird comfortably. Don't worry if the body comes up above the rim. Cover with clingfilm (plastic wrap) and puncture 4 times. Cook on Full for 4 minutes per 450 g/1 lb. Remove from the oven and carefully turn the bird over so that the breast is now uppermost. Brush thickly with a baste, using a fat-based one if the bird is plain and a non-fat one if the turkey is self-basting. Cover as before and cook on Full for a further 4 minutes per 450 g/1 lb. Transfer to a carving dish and cover with foil. Leave to stand for 15 minutes, then carve.

Spanish Turkey

Serves 4

30 ml/2 tbsp olive oil

4 pieces boned turkey breast, 175 g/6 oz each

1 onion, chopped

12 stuffed olives, chopped

2 hard-boiled (hard-cooked) eggs (pages 98–9), shelled and chopped

30 ml/2 tbsp chopped gherkins (cornichons)

2 tomatoes, thinly sliced

Heat the oil in a deep 20 cm/8 in diameter dish, uncovered, on Full for 1 minute. Add the turkey and toss well in the oil to coat both sides thoroughly. Combine the onion, olives, eggs and gherkins and spoon equally on to the turkey. Garnish with the tomato slices. Cover with clingfilm (plastic wrap) and slit it twice to allow steam to escape. Cook on Full for 15 minutes, turning the dish five times. Allow to stand for 5 minutes before serving.

Turkey Tacos

Serves 4

For the tacos:

450 g/1 lb/4 cups minced turkey

1 small onion, chopped

2 garlic cloves, crushed

5 ml/1 tsp cumin seeds, ground if preferred

2.5–5 ml/½–1 tsp chilli powder

30 ml/2 tbsp chopped coriander (cilantro) leaves

5 ml/1 tsp salt

60 ml/4 tbsp water

4 large bought tortillas

Shredded lettuce

For the avocado garnish:

1 large ripe avocado

15–20 ml/3–4 tsp bought hot salsa

Juice of 1 lime

Salt

60 ml/4 tbsp soured (dairy sour) cream

To make the tacos, cover the base of a 20 cm/8 in diameter dish with the turkey. Cover with a plate and cook on Full for 6 minutes. Break down the grains of meat with a fork. Stir in all the remaining ingredients except the tortillas and lettuce. Cover with clingfilm (plastic wrap) and slit it twice to allow steam to escape. Cook on Full for 8 minutes, turning the dish four times. Allow to stand for 4 minutes. Stir thoroughly. Pile equal amounts of the turkey mixture on the tortillas, add some lettuce and roll up. Transfer to a dish and keep warm.

To make the avocado dressing, halve the avocado, scoop out the flesh and mash finely. Stir in the salsa, lime juice and salt. Transfer the tacos to four warmed plates, top each with the avocado mixture and 15 ml/1 tbsp soured cream. Eat straight away.

Pancake Tacos

Serves 4

Prepare as for Turkey Tacos, but substitute four large home-made pancakes for the bought tortillas.

Turkey Loaf

Serves 4

450 g/1 lb raw minced (ground) turkey

1 garlic clove, crushed

30 ml/2 tbsp plain (all-purpose) flour

2 large eggs, beaten

10 ml/2 tsp salt

10 ml/2 tsp dried thyme

5 ml/1 tsp Worcestershire sauce

20 ml/4 tsp ground nutmeg

Jacket Potatoes

Cooked cauliflower

Cheese Sauce

Mix together the turkey, garlic, flour, eggs, salt, thyme, Worcestershire sauce and nutmeg. With damp hands, shape into a 15 cm/6 in loaf. Transfer to a deep dish, cover with clingfilm (plastic wrap) and slit it twice to allow steam to escape. Cook on Full for 9 minutes. Allow to stand for 5 minutes. Slice into four portions and serve with jacket potatoes and cauliflower, coated with cheese sauce and browned conventionally under the grill (broiler).

Anglo-Madras Turkey Curry

Serves 4

A useful recipe to use up Christmas turkey leftovers.

30 ml/2 tbsp corn or sunflower oil

1 large onion, very thinly sliced

1 garlic clove, crushed

30 ml/2 tbsp raisins

30 ml/2 tbsp desiccated (shredded) coconut

25 ml/1½ tbsp plain (all-purpose) flour

20 ml/4 tsp hot curry powder

300 ml/½ pt/1¼ cups boiling water

30 ml/2 tbsp single (light) cream

2.5 ml/½ tsp salt

Juice of ½ lemon

350 g/12 oz/3 cups cold cooked turkey, cubed

Indian bread, mixed salad and chutney, to serve

Put the oil in a 1.5 litre/2½ pt/6 cup dish with the onion, garlic, raisins and coconut. Mix well. Cook, uncovered, on Full for 3 minutes. Mix in the flour, curry powder, water, cream, salt, lemon juice and turkey. Cover with a plate and cook on Full for 6–7 minutes, stirring twice, until the curry is thickened and bubbling. Allow to stand for 3 minutes. Stir round and serve with Indian bread, salad and chutney.

Fruited Turkey Curry

Serves 4

30 ml/2 tbsp butter or margarine

10 ml/2 tsp olive oil

2 onions, chopped

15 ml/1 tbsp mild curry powder

30 ml/2 tbsp plain (all-purpose) flour

150 ml/¼ pt/2/3 cup single (light) cream

90 ml/6 tbsp Greek-style plain yoghurt

1 garlic clove, crushed

30 ml/2 tbsp tomato purée (paste)

5 ml/1 tsp garam masala

5 ml/1 tsp salt

Juice of 1 small lime

4 eating (dessert) apples, peeled, cored, quartered and thinly sliced

30 ml/2 tbsp any fruit chutney

450 g/1 lb/4 cups cold cooked turkey, cubed

Put the butter or margarine and oil in a 25 cm/10 in diameter casserole dish (Dutch oven). Heat, uncovered, on Full for 1½ minutes. Mix in the onions. Cook, uncovered, on Full for 3 minutes, stirring twice. Stir in the curry powder, flour, cream and yoghurt. Cook, uncovered, on Full for 2 minutes. Add all the remaining ingredients. Cover with a plate and cook on Full for 12–14 minutes, stirring every 5 minutes, until piping hot.

Bread and Butter Turkey Pie

Serves 4

75 g/3 oz/3/8 cup butter or margarine

60 ml/4 tbsp grated Parmesan cheese

2.5 ml/½ tsp dried thyme

1.5 ml/¼ tsp dried sage

5 ml/1 tsp grated lemon peel

4 large slices white or brown bread

1 onion, chopped

50 g/2 oz mushrooms, sliced

45 ml/3 tbsp plain (all-purpose) flour

300 ml/½ pt/1¼ cups warm chicken stock

15 ml/1 tbsp lemon juice

45 ml/3 tbsp single (light) cream

225 g/8 oz/2 cups cold cooked chicken, cubed

Salt and freshly ground black pepper

Cream half the butter or margarine with the cheese, thyme, sage and lemon peel. Spread over the bread, then cut each slice into four triangles. Put the remaining butter or margarine in a deep 20 cm/8 in diameter dish. Heat, uncovered, on Full for 1½ minutes. Add the onion and mushrooms. Cook, uncovered, on Full for 3 minutes, stirring twice. Mix in the flour, then gradually blend in the stock, lemon juice and cream. Stir in the chicken and season to taste. Cover with a plate and heat on Full for 8 minutes, stirring three times, until piping hot. Remove from the microwave. Top with the buttered bread triangles and brown under a hot grill (broiler).

Turkey and Rice Casserole with Stuffing

Serves 4–5

225 g/8 oz/1 cup easy-cook long-grain rice

300 ml/10 fl oz/1 can condensed cream of mushroom soup

300 ml/½ pt/1¼ cups boiling water

225 g/8 oz/2 cups sweetcorn (corn)

50 g/2 oz/½ cup chopped unsalted nuts

175 g/6 oz/1½ cups cooked turkey, diced

50 g/2 oz cold stuffing, cubed

Coleslaw, to serve

Put all the ingredients except the stuffing in a 1.75 litre/3 pt/7½ cup dish. Mix thoroughly. Cover with clingfilm (plastic wrap) and slit it twice to allow steam to escape. Cook on Full for 25 minutes. Uncover and stir with a fork to fluff up the rice. Top with the cold stuffing. Cover with a plate and cook on Full for 2 minutes. Allow to stand for 4 minutes. Fluff up again and eat with coleslaw.

Turkey Breast with Orange Glaze

Serves 4–6

For small families who want a festive meal with minimal leftovers.

40 g/1½ oz/3 tbsp butter

15 ml/1 tbsp tomato ketchup (catsup)

10 ml/2 tsp black treacle (molasses)

5 ml/1 tsp paprika

5 ml/1 tsp Worcestershire sauce

Finely grated peel of 1 satsuma or clementine

A pinch of ground cloves

1.5 ml/¼ tsp ground cinnamon

1 whole turkey breast, about 1 kg/2¼ lb

Thoroughly combine all the ingredients except the turkey in a dish. Heat, uncovered, on Defrost for 1 minute. Place the turkey breast in a 25 cm/10 in diameter dish (Dutch oven) and brush with half the baste. Cover with clingfilm (plastic wrap) and slit it twice to allow steam to escape. Cook on Full for 10 minutes. Turn the turkey breast over and brush with the remaining baste. Cover as before and cook on Full for a further 10 minutes, turning the dish three times. Allow to stand for 7–10 minutes before carving.

Sweet and Sour Duck

Serves 4

1 duck, about 2.25 kg/5 lb, washed and dried

45 ml/3 tbsp mango chutney

Bean sprouts

175 g/6 oz/¾ cup brown rice, boiled

Stand the duck upside-down on an upturned tea plate standing in a 25 cm/10 in diameter casserole dish (Dutch oven). Cover with clingfilm (plastic wrap) and slit it twice to allow steam to escape. Cook on Full for 20 minutes. Uncover and carefully pour off the fat and juices. Turn the duck over and spread the breast with the chutney. Cover as before and cook on Full for a further 20 minutes. Cut into four portions and serve with bean sprouts and the rice.

Canton Duck

Serves 4

45 ml/3 tbsp smooth apricot jam (conserve)

30 ml/2 tbsp Chinese rice wine

10 ml/2 tsp mild made mustard

5 ml/1 tsp lemon juice

10 ml/2 tsp soy sauce

1 duck, about 2.25 kg/5 lb, washed and dried

Put the apricot jam, rice wine, mustard, lemon juice and soy sauce in a small basin. Heat on Full for 1–1½ minutes, stirring twice. Stand the duck upside-down on an upturned tea plate standing in a 25 cm/10 in diameter casserole dish (Dutch oven). Cover with clingfilm (plastic wrap) and slit it twice to allow steam to escape. Cook on Full for 20 minutes. Uncover and carefully pour off the fat and juices. Turn the duck over and spread the breast with the apricot baste. Cover as before and cook on Full for 20 minutes. Cut into four portions and serve.

Serves 4

A high-class luxury, easily prepared in the microwave in a fraction of the time it would normally take. Garnish with watercress and fresh orange slices for a party centrepiece.

1 duck, about 2.25 kg/5 lb, washed and dried

For the sauce:

Finely grated peel of 1 large orange

Juice of 2 oranges

30 ml/2 tbsp fine-shred lemon marmalade

15 ml/1 tbsp redcurrant jelly (clear conserve)

30 ml/2 tbsp orange liqueur

5 ml/1 tsp soy sauce

10 ml/2 tsp cornflour (cornstarch)

Stand the duck upside-down on an upturned tea plate standing in a 25 cm/10 in diameter casserole dish (Dutch oven). Cover with clingfilm (plastic wrap) and slit it twice to allow steam to escape. Cook on Full for 20 minutes. Uncover and carefully pour off the fat and juices. Turn the duck over. Cover as before and cook on Full for 20 minutes. Cut into four portions, transfer to a serving dish and keep hot. Skim the fat from the cooking juices.

To make the sauce, place all the ingredients except the cornflour in a measuring jug. Add the skimmed cooking juices. Make up to 300 ml/½ pt/1¼ cups with hot water. Mix the cornflour to a thin paste with a few spoonfuls of cold water. Add to the jug and mix thoroughly. Cook, uncovered, on Full for 4 minutes, stirring three times. Pour over the duck and serve straight away.

French-style Duck

Serves 4

1 duck, about 2.25 kg/5 lb, washed and dried

12 stoned (pitted) prunes

1 celery stalk, finely chopped

2 garlic cloves, crushed

For the sauce:

300 ml/½ pt/1¼ cups dry cider

5 ml/1 tsp salt

10 ml/2 tsp tomato purée (paste)

30 ml/2 tbsp crème fraîche

15 ml/1 tbsp cornflour (cornstarch)

Boiled tagliatelle, to serve

Stand the duck upside-down on an upturned tea plate standing in a 25 cm/10 in diameter casserole dish (Dutch oven). Scatter the prunes, celery and garlic around the duck. Cover the dish with clingfilm (plastic wrap) and slit it twice to allow steam to escape. Cook on Full for 20 minutes. Uncover and carefully pour off and reserve the fat and juices. Turn the duck over. Cover as before and cook on Full for 20 minutes. Cut into four portions, transfer to a serving dish and keep hot. Skim the fat from the cooking juices.

To make the sauce, place the cider in a measuring jug. Whisk in the salt, tomato purée, crème fraîche, the skimmed cooking juices and cornflour. Cook, uncovered, on Full for 4–5 minutes until thickened and bubbling, whisking every minute. Pour over the duck and prunes and accompany with tagliatelle.

Roasting Boned and Rolled Joints of Meat

Place the joint, skin side up, on a special microwave trivet standing in a large dish. Cover with a piece of clingfilm (plastic wrap). For every 450 g/1 lb allow the following cooking times:

- Pork – 9 minutes
- Ham – 9 minutes
- Lamb – 9 minutes
- Beef – 6–8 minutes

Turn the dish every 5 minutes for even cooking, protecting your hands with oven gloves. Allow to rest for 5–6 minutes half-way through the roasting time. At the end of cooking, transfer the joint to a carving board and cover with a double thickness of foil. Allow to rest for 5–8 minutes, depending on its size, before carving.

Sweet and Sour Pork Chops with Orange and Lime

Serves 4

4 pork chops, 175 g/6 oz each after trimming

60 ml/4 tbsp tomato ketchup (catsup)

15 ml/1 tbsp teriyaki sauce

20 ml/4 tsp malt vinegar

5 ml/1 tsp finely grated lime peel

Juice of 1 orange

1 garlic clove, crushed (optional)

350 g/12 oz/1½ cups brown rice, boiled

Arrange the chops in a deep 25 cm/10 in diameter dish. Beat together all the remaining ingredients except the rice and spoon over the chops. Cover with clingfilm (plastic wrap) and slit it twice to allow steam to escape. Cook on Full for 12 minutes, turning the dish four times. Allow to stand for 5 minutes before serving with the brown rice.

Meat Loaf

Serves 8–10

A tried and trusted versatile family terrine. It is excellent when served hot, cut into wedges with gravy or Portugese Sauce or Rustic Tomato Sauce and accompanied with Creamed Potatoes or macaroni cheese and assorted vegetables. Alternatively, eat it cold with a rich mayonnaise or salad dressing and salad. For sandwiches, slice thinly and use as a filling with lettuce, chopped spring onions (scallions) and tomatoes or, served with baby gherkins (cornichons) and granary bread, it has the makings of a classic French-style starter.

125 g/4¾ oz/3½ slices light-textured white bread
450 g/1 lb lean minced (ground) beef
450 g/1 lb/4 cups minced (ground) turkey
10 ml/2 tsp salt
3 garlic cloves, crushed
4 large eggs, beaten
10 ml/2 tsp Worcestershire sauce
10 ml/2 tsp dark soy sauce
10 ml/2 tsp made mustard

Lightly grease a deep 23 cm/9 in diameter dish. Crumb the bread in a food processor. Add all the remaining ingredients and pulse the machine until the mixture is just combined. (Avoid over-mixing as the loaf will be heavy and dense.) Spread into the prepared dish. Push a baby jam (conserve) jar or straight-sided egg cup into the centre so that the meat mixture forms a ring. Cover with clingfilm (plastic wrap) and slit it twice to allow steam to escape. Cook on Full for 18 minutes, turning the dish twice. The loaf will shrink away from sides of dish. Leave to stand for 5 minutes if serving hot.

Turkey and Sausagemeat Terrine

Serves 8–10

Prepare as for Meat Loaf, but substitute 450 g/1 lb beef or pork sausagemeat for the minced (ground) beef. Cook on Full for 18 minutes instead of 20 minutes.

Pork Chops with Zippy Dressing

Serves 4

4 pork chops, 175 g/6 oz each after trimming
30 ml/2 tbsp butter or margarine
5 ml/1 tsp paprika
5 ml/1 tsp soy sauce
5 ml/1 tsp Worcestershire sauce

Arrange the chops in a deep 25 cm/10 in diameter dish. Melt the butter or margarine on Defrost for 1½ minutes. Beat in the remaining ingredients and pour over the chops. Cover with clingfilm (plastic wrap) and slit it twice to allow steam to escape. Cook on Full for 9 minutes, turning the dish four times. Allow to stand for 4 minutes.

Hawaiian Pork and Pineapple Casserole

Serves 6

Delicacy, tenderness and a fine flavour characterise this meat and fruit recipe from the tropical island of Hawaii.

15 ml/1 tbsp groundnut (peanut) oil

1 onion, finely chopped

2 garlic cloves, crushed

900 g/2 lb pork fillet, cubed

15 ml/1 tbsp cornflour (cornstarch)

400 g/14 oz/3½ cups canned crushed pineapple in natural juice

45 ml/3 tbsp soy sauce

5 ml//1 tsp ground ginger

Freshly ground black pepper

Brush the oil over the base and sides of a deep 23 cm/9 in diameter dish. Add the onion and garlic and cook, uncovered, on Full for 3 minutes. Stir in the pork, cornflour, pineapple and juice, soy sauce and ginger. Season to taste with pepper. Arrange in a ring round the inside edge of the dish, leaving a small hollow in the centre. Cover with clingfilm (plastic wrap) and slit it twice to allow steam to escape. Cook on Full for 16 minutes, turning the dish four times. Allow to stand for 5 minutes, then stir before serving.

Hawaiian Gammon and Pineapple Casserole

Serves 6

Prepare as for Hawaiian Pork and Pineapple Casserole, but substitute unsmoked and mild gammon cubes for the pork.

Festive Gammon

Serves 10–12

Ideal for a Christmas or New Year buffet, gammon cooked in the microwave is moist and succulent and carves beautifully. This is the maximum size for a satisfactory result.

Gammon joint, maximum weight 2.5 kg/5½ lb

50 g/2 oz/1 cup browned breadcrumbs

Whole cloves

The joint is first boiled conventionally to decrease saltiness. Place the gammon in a large saucepan, cover with cold water, bring to the boil and drain. Repeat. Weigh the drained joint and allow 8 minutes cooking time on Full per 450 g/1 lb. Either stand the joint directly on the glass tray inside the microwave or put it in a large shallow dish. If there is a narrow end, wrap it in a piece of foil to prevent overcooking. Cover the gammon with kitchen paper and cook for half the cooking time. Allow to stand in the microwave for 30 minutes. Remove the foil, if used, turn the joint over and cover with kitchen paper. Complete the cooking and leave to stand for a further 30 minutes. Transfer to a board. Strip off the skin, score the fat into diamonds, then sprinkle with the crumbs. Stud each diamond with a clove.

Glazed Gala Gammon

Serves 10–12

Gammon joint, maximum weight 2.5 kg/5½ lb

50 g/2 oz/1 cup browned breadcrumbs

Whole cloves

60 ml/4 tbsp demerara sugar

10 ml/2 tsp mustard powder

60 ml/4 tbsp butter or margarine, melted

5 ml/1 tsp Worcestershire sauce

30 ml/2 tbsp white grape juice

Cocktail cherries

Prepare as for Festive Gammon, but stud each alternate diamond with a clove. To make the glaze, mix together the sugar, mustard, butter or margarine, Worcestershire sauce and grape juice. Transfer the gammon to a roasting tin and cover the fat with the glaze. Cook the joint conventionally at 190°C/375°F/gas mark 5 for 25–30 minutes until the fat is golden brown. Stud the remaining diamonds of fat with cocktail cherries speared on to cocktail sticks (toothpicks).

Paella with Spanish Salami

Serves 6

Prepare as for Paella, but substitute coarsely chopped salami for the chicken.

Swedish-style Meatballs

Serves 4

Known as kottbullar, this is one of Sweden's national dishes, where it is served with boiled potatoes, cranberry sauce, gravy and a mixed salad.

75 g/3 oz/1½ cups fresh white breadcrumbs
1 onion, finely chopped
225 g/8 oz/2 cups lean minced (ground) pork
225 g/8 oz/2 cups minced (ground) beef
1 large egg
2.5 ml/½ tsp salt
175 ml/6 fl oz/1 small can evaporated milk
2.5 ml/½ tsp ground allspice
25 g/1 oz/2 tbsp margarine

Thoroughly combine all the ingredients except the margarine. Shape into 12 even-sized balls. Heat a microwave browning dish as directed either on page 14 or in the instruction book supplied with your dish or microwave. Add the margarine and, with hands protected by oven gloves, swirl the dish until the base is completely covered. At this point it will also sizzle. Add the meatballs and turn immediately to brown all over. Cover with clingfilm (plastic wrap) and slit it twice to allow steam to escape. Cook on Full for 9½ minutes, turning the dish four times. Allow to stand for 3 minutes before serving.

Roast Pork with Crackling

A surprisingly crisp skin on the pork, due to the meat's long cooking time.

Choose a piece of leg, allowing 175 g/6 oz per person. Score the skin deeply with a knife and sprinkle thickly with salt and more lightly with paprika. Place the joint, skin side up, on a special microwave trivet standing in a large dish. Cover with a piece of baking parchment. Open roast like this, allowing 9 minutes for every 450 g/1 lb. Turn the dish every 5 minutes for even cooking, protecting your hands with oven gloves. Allow to rest for 6 minutes half-way through the cooking time. At the end of cooking, transfer the joint to a carving board and cover with a double thickness of foil. Allow to stand for 8 minutes before carving and serve with vegetables and Sage and Onion Stuffing.

Roast Pork with Honey

Prepare as for Roast Pork with Crackling, but brush with a baste made from 90 ml/6 tbsp dark clear honey mixed with a 20 ml/generous 1 tbsp made mustard and 10 ml/2 tsp Worcestershire sauce before sprinkling with salt and paprika.

Pork Chops with Red Cabbage

Serves 4

A winter affair, when jars and cans of red cabbage fill the shelves for Christmas. Eat with Creamed Potatoes and mashed parsnip.

450 g/1 lb cooked red cabbage

4 tomatoes, blanched, skinned and chopped

10 ml/2 tsp salt

4 pork chops, 175 g/6 oz each after trimming

10 ml/2 tsp soy sauce

2.5 ml/½ tsp garlic salt

2.5 ml/½ tsp paprika

15 ml/1 tbsp dark soft brown sugar

Arrange the cabbage over the base of a 20 cm/8 in diameter casserole dish (Dutch oven). Mix in the tomatoes and salt and place the chops on top. Pour the soy sauce over and sprinkle with the remaining ingredients. Cover with clingfilm (plastic wrap) and slit it twice to allow steam to escape. Cook on Full for 15 minutes, turning the dish four times. Allow to stand for 4 minutes before serving.

Roman-style Pork Fillets

Serves 4

15 ml/1 tbsp olive oil

1 small onion, chopped

1 garlic clove, crushed

4 slices pork fillet, 125 g/4 oz each, beaten until very thin

60 ml/4 tbsp tomato juice

5 ml/1 tsp dried oregano

125 g/4 oz Mozzarella cheese, sliced

30 ml/2 tbsp capers

Polenta

Pour the oil into a deep 25 cm/10 in diameter dish. Heat on Full for 1 minute. Stir in the onion and garlic. Cook, uncovered, on Full for 4 minutes, stirring twice. Add the pork to the dish in single layer. Cook, uncovered, on Full for 2 minutes. Turn over and cook for a further 2 minutes. Sprinkle with the tomato juice and oregano, top with the Mozzarella slices, then stud with the capers. Cover with clingfilm (plastic wrap) and slit it twice to allow steam to escape. Cook on Full for 2–3 minutes or until the cheese is just melting. Allow to stand for 1 minute before serving with polenta.

Pork Fillet and Vegetable Casserole

Serves 6–8

15 ml/1 tbsp sunflower or corn oil

1 onion, grated

2 garlic cloves, crushed

675 g/1½ lb pork fillet, cut into 1.5 cm/¾ in slices

30 ml/2 tbsp plain (all-purpose) flour

5 ml/1 tsp dried marjoram

5 ml/1 tsp finely grated orange peel

200 g/7 oz/1¾ cups canned or thawed frozen mixed peas and carrots

200 g/7 oz/1½ cups sweetcorn (corn)

300 ml/½ pt/1¼ cups rosé wine

150 ml/¼ pt/2/3 cup hot water

5 ml/1 tsp salt

Pour the oil into a 2 litre/3½ pt/8½ cup casserole dish (Dutch oven). Heat, uncovered, on Full for 1 minute. Mix in the onion and garlic. Cook, uncovered, on Full for 4 minutes, stirring twice. Add the pork. Cover the dish with a plate and cook on Full for 4 minutes. Mix in the flour, making sure the pieces of meat are well coated. Add all remaining ingredients except the salt. Cover with clingfilm (plastic wrap) and slit it twice to allow steam to escape. Cook on Full for 17 minutes, turning the dish four times. Allow to stand for 5 minutes before seasoning with the salt and serving.

Chilli Pork Chops

Serves 4

4 pork spare rib chops, 225 g/8 oz each, fat removed

10 ml/2 tsp chilli or Cajun seasoning

5 ml/1 tsp garlic powder

400 g/14 oz/1 large can red kidney beans, drained

400 g/14 oz/1 large can chopped tomatoes

30 ml/2 tbsp chopped fresh coriander (cilantro)

2.5 ml/½ tsp salt

Arrange the chops in a deep 30 cm/12 in diameter dish. Sprinkle with the seasoning and garlic powder. Cover with clingfilm (plastic wrap) and slit it twice to allow steam to escape. Cook on Full for 8 minutes, turning the dish twice. Uncover and spread with the beans and tomatoes with their juice. Sprinkle with the coriander and salt. Cover as before and cook on Full for 15 minutes, turning 3 times. Allow to stand for 5 minutes before serving.

Pork with Chutney and Mandarins

Serves 4

4 pork spare rib chops, 225 g/8 oz each, fat removed

350 g/12 oz/1 large can mandarin segments in light syrup

5 ml/1 tsp paprika

20 ml/4 tsp soy sauce

45 ml/3 tbsp fruit chutney, chopped if necessary

2 garlic cloves, crushed

Curried Rice

Arrange the chops in a deep 30 cm/12 in diameter dish. Drain the mandarins, reserving 30 ml/2 tbsp of the syrup, and divide the fruit over the chops. Beat the reserved syrup with the remaining ingredients except the rice and spoon over the mandarins. Cover with clingfilm (plastic wrap) and slit it twice to allow steam to escape. Cook on Full for 20 minutes, turning the dish four times. Allow to stand for 5 minutes, then serve with the rice.

'Barbecued' Ribs

Serves 4

1 kg/2¼ lb meaty pork sheet ribs or spare ribs

50 g/2 oz/¼ cup butter or margarine

15 ml/1 tbsp tomato ketchup (catsup)

10 ml/2 tsp soy sauce

5 ml/1 tsp paprika

1 garlic clove, crushed

5 ml/1 tsp hot chilli sauce

Wash and dry the pork and separate into individual ribs. Arrange in the largest round shallow dish that will fit comfortably in the microwave, with the narrow part of each rib pointing towards the centre. Cover with clingfilm (plastic wrap) and slit it twice to allow steam to escape. Cook on Full for 10 minutes, turning the dish three times. To make the baste, combine the remaining ingredients in a bowl and warm, uncovered, on Defrost for 2 minutes. Uncover the ribs and carefully pour off the fat. Brush with about half the the baste. Cook, uncovered, on Full for 3 minutes. Turn over with tongs and brush with the remaining baste. Cook, uncovered, on Full for 2 minutes. Allow to stand for 3 minutes before serving.

Ham-wrapped Chicory in Cheese Sauce

Serves 4

Called chicorées au jambon in Belgium, its country of origin. The silvery-white vegetable wrapped in ham and enveloped in a simple cheese sauce is a gastonomic masterpiece.

8 heads chicory (Belgian endive), about 1 kg/2¼ lb in all

150 ml/¼ pt/2/3 cup boiling water

15 ml/1 tbsp lemon juice

8 large slices cooked ham

600 ml/1 pt/2½ cups milk

50 g/2 oz/¼ cup butter or margarine

45 ml/3 tbsp plain (all-purpose) flour

175 g/6 oz/1½ cups Edam cheese, grated

Salt and freshly ground pepper

Chips (fries), to serve

Trim the chicory, removing any bruised or damaged outer leaves, and cut out a cone-shaped piece from the base of each to prevent a bitter taste. Arrange the heads like spokes of a wheel in a deep 30 cm/12 in diameter dish. Coat with the water and lemon juice. Cover with clingfilm (plastic wrap) and slit it twice to allow steam to escape. Cook on Full for 14 minutes, turning the dish twice. Allow to stand for 5 minutes, then drain thoroughly. Wash and dry the dish. When the chicory is lukewarm, wrap a ham slice round each and return to the dish. Place the milk in a jug and heat, uncovered, on Full for 3 minutes. Put butter or margarine into a 1.2 litre/2 pt/5 cup dish and melt on Full for 1 minute. Stir in the flour, then gradually whisk in the hot milk. Cook, uncovered, on Full for 5–6 minutes, whisking every minute to ensure smoothness, until the sauce is bubbly and thickened. Mix in the cheese and season to taste. Pour evenly over the chicory and ham. Cover with a plate and reheat on Full for 3 minutes. Allow to stand for 3 minutes. Brown conventionally under a hot grill (broiler), if liked, then serve with chips.

Pork Ribs in Sticky Orange Barbecue Sauce

Serves 4

1 kg/2¼ lb meaty pork sheet ribs or spare ribs

30 ml/2 tbsp lemon juice

30 ml/2 tbsp soy sauce

5 ml/1 tsp Japanese wasabi powder

15 ml/1 tbsp Worcestershire sauce

300 ml/½ pt/1¼ cups freshly squeezed orange juice

30 ml/2 tbsp dark orange marmalade

10 ml/2 tsp made mustard

1 garlic clove, crushed

Chinese noodles, boiled, to serve

A few orange wedges, to garnish

Place the ribs in a large shallow dish. Cover with clingfilm (plastic wrap) and slit it twice to allow steam to escape. Cook on Full for 7 minutes, turning the dish twice. Uncover and carefully pour off the fat. Beat together the remaining ingredients except the noodles and pour over the ribs. Cover loosely with kitchen paper and cook on Full for 20 minutes, turning the dish four times and basting with sauce each time. Eat with boiled Chinese noodles and orange wedges served separately.

Steak and Mushroom Pudding

Serves 4

This old English treasure works like a dream in the microwave, with the suet crust pastry (paste) behaving exactly as it should. The trick is to use precooked meat, such as a home-made stew or canned meat, because cubes of raw meat have a tendency to toughen in the microwave when cooked with liquid.

For the pastry:

175 g/6 oz/1½ cups self-raising (self-rising) flour

2.5 ml/½ tsp salt

50 g/2 oz/½ cup shredded beef or vegetarian suet

90 ml/6 tbsp cold water

For the filling:

450 g/1 lb stewed meat with gravy

125 g/4 oz button mushrooms

To make the pastry, sift the flour and salt into bowl and toss in the suet. Using a fork, stir in enough of the water to make a soft but pliable dough. Knead lightly until smooth, then roll out on a floured surface to a 30 cm/12 in round. Cut out a wedge-shaped quarter and reserve for the lid. Throughly grease a 900 ml/1½ pt/3¾ cup pudding basin and line with the pastry, easing it over the base and sides until it reaches the inner rim at the top of the basin and pressing out any wrinkles with your fingertips. Seal the joins by pinching them together with dampened fingers.

To make the filling, heat together the stewed meat and mushrooms, either in the microwave or conventionally. Allow to cool. Spoon into the pastry-lined basin. Roll out the reserved pastry to make a lid, dampen the edge and place on the lining pastry, pinching them together to seal. Cover with clingfilm (plastic wrap) and slit it twice to allow steam to escape. Cook on Full for 7 minutes until the pastry is well risen. Allow to stand for 3 minutes, then spoon out on to plates to serve.

Steak and Kidney Pudding

Serves 4

Prepare as for Steak and Mushroom Pudding, but use 450 g/1 lb mixed stewed steak and kidney.

Steak and Chestnut Pudding

Serves 4

Prepare as for Steak and Mushroom Pudding, but substitute whole chestnuts for the button mushrooms.

Steak and Pickled Walnut Pudding with Prunes

Serves 4

Prepare as for Steak and Mushroom Pudding, but substitute 4 pickled walnuts, quartered, and 8 stoned (pitted) prunes for the mushrooms.

South American 'Chopped' Meat

Serves 4

2 onions, finely chopped or grated

275 g/10 oz peeled pumpkin, butternut squash or unpeeled courgettes (zucchini), diced

1 large tomato, blanched, skinned and chopped

450 g/1 lb/4 cups coarsely minced (ground) beef

5–10 ml/1–2 tsp salt

Brazilian Rice

Put the vegetables and mince in a 20 cm/8 inch diameter casserole dish (Dutch oven). Cover with clingfilm (plastic wrap) and slit it twice to allow steam to escape. Cook on Full for 10 minutes, turning the dish three times. Uncover and mash thoroughly to break up the meat. Cover with a plate and cook on Full for 5 minutes, stirring once. Allow to stand for 3 minutes and season with the salt. The meat will be a fairly loose consistency in its unthickened gravy. Serve with Brazilian rice.

Brazilian 'Chopped' Meat with Eggs and Olives

Serves 4

Prepare as for South American Chopped Meat, but omit the pumpkin, squash or courgettes (zucchini). Add 60 ml/4 tbsp stock to the meat mixture. Reduce the initial cooking time to 7 minutes. After standing, stir in 3 hard-boiled (hard-cooked) egg wedges and 12 stoned (pitted) green olives.

The Reuben Sandwich

Serves 2

As any North American will testify, the open Reuben Sandwich is a feast of a meal, produced by delis from New York to California.

2 large slices brown or rye bread
Mayonnaise
175 g/6 oz salt beef, pastrami or brisket, thinly sliced
175 g/6 oz drained sauerkraut
4 large thin slices Gruyère (Swiss) or Emmental cheese

Spread the bread with mayonnaise and place the slices side by side on a large plate. Heat, uncovered, on Defrost for 1½ minutes. Cover each evenly with the beef and top with the sauerkraut, pressing it down lightly with a spatula. Cover with the cheese. Cook on Full for 1½ –2 minutes until the cheese melts. Eat straight away.

Beef Chow Mein

Serves 4

Prepare as for Chicken Chow Mein, but substitute beef for the chicken.

Beef Chop Suey

Serves 4

Prepare as for Chicken Chop Suey, but substitute beef for the chicken.

Aubergine and Beef Casserole

Serves 6

This Louisiana speciality is a treat for one and all and is relished by the locals.

4 aubergines (eggplants)

10 ml/2 tsp salt

45 ml/3 tbsp boiling water

1 onion, finely grated

450 g/1 lb/4 cups lean minced (ground) beef

75 g/3 oz/1½ cups fresh white breadcrumbs

1.5–2.5 ml/¼–½ tsp hot pepper sauce

Salt and freshly ground pepper

25 g/1 oz/2 tbsp butter

250 g/8 oz/2¼ cups American long-grain rice, boiled

Top, tail and peel the aubergines and cube the flesh. Put into a large bowl or dish and mix in the salt and boiling water. Cover with clingfilm (plastic wrap) and slit it twice to allow steam to escape. Cook on Full for 14 minutes. Allow to stand for 2 minutes. Drain thoroughly, then place in a blender or food processor and process to a purée. Thoroughly grease a shallow dish. Mix together the aubergine purée, onion, beef, half the breadcrumbs, the pepper sauce and salt and freshly ground black pepper to taste. Spread into the casserole. Sprinkle with the remaining breadcrumbs, then dot with flakes of butter. Cook, uncovered, on Full for 10 minutes. Flash briefly under a hot grill (broiler) before serving, if liked, to crisp the top. Serve with the rice.

Meatball Curry

Serves 8

675 g/1½ lb/6 cups lean minced (ground) beef

50 g/2 oz/1 cup fresh white breadcrumbs

1 garlic clove, crushed

1 large egg, beaten

300 ml/10 fl oz/1 can condensed tomato soup

6 tomatoes

10 ml/2 tsp soy sauce

15–30 ml/1–2 tbsp mild curry powder

15 ml/1 tbsp tomato purée (paste)

1 beef stock cube

75 ml/5 tbsp mango chutney

Boiled rice or mashed potato, to serve

Mix together the beef, breadcrumbs, garlic and egg. Shape into 16 balls and arrange round the edge of a deep 25 cm/10 in diameter dish. Mix together the remaining ingredients and spoon over the meatballs. Cover with clingfilm (plastic wrap) and slit it twice to allow steam to escape. Cook on Full for 18 minutes, turning the dish four times. Allow to stand for 5 minutes. Uncover and baste the meatballs with the sauce. Leave uncovered and reheat on Full for a further 1½–2 minutes. Serve with boiled rice or mashed potato.

Italian Meatballs

Serves 4

15 ml/2 tbsp olive oil

1 onion, grated

2 garlic cloves, crushed

450 g/1 lb/4 cups lean minced (ground) beef

75 ml/5 tbsp fresh white breadcrumbs

1 egg, beaten

10 ml/2 tsp salt

400 g/14 oz/1¾ cups passata (sieved tomatoes)

10 ml/2 tsp dark soft brown sugar

5 ml/1 tsp dried basil or oregano

Pour the oil into a deep 20 cm/8 in diameter dish. Add the onion and garlic. Cook, uncovered, on Full for 4 minutes. Combine the meat with the breadcrumbs, egg and half the salt. Shape into 12 small balls. Add to the dish and cook, uncovered, on Full for 5 minutes, turning the meatballs half-way through the cooking time. Stand while mixing together the passata, sugar, oregano and remaining salt. Pour over the meatballs. Cover with clingfilm (plastic wrap) and slit it twice to allow steam to escape. Cook on Full for 10 minutes, turning the dish three times. Allow to stand for 3 minutes before serving.

Speedy Paprika Meatballs

Serves 4–6

This is good with plain boiled potatoes, or microwaved chips (fries) if you're really in a hurry!

450 g/1 lb/4 cups lean minced (ground) beef

50 g/2 oz/1 cup fresh white breadcrumbs

1 garlic clove, crushed

1 large egg, beaten

300 ml/½ pt/1¼ cups passata (sieved tomatoes)

300 ml/½ pt/1¼ cups boiling water

30 ml/2 tbsp dried red and green (bell) pepper flakes

10 ml/2 tsp paprika

5 ml/1 tsp caraway seeds (optional)

10 ml/2 tsp dark soft brown sugar

5 ml/1 tsp salt

150 ml/5 oz/2/3 cup soured (dairy sour) cream

Mix together the meat, breadcrumbs, garlic and egg. Shape into 12 balls. Arrange round the edge of a deep 20 cm/8 in diameter dish. Combine the passata with the water. Stir in the pepper flakes, paprika, caraway seeds, if using, and sugar. Spoon over the meatballs. Cover with clingfilm (plastic wrap) and slit it twice to allow steam to escape. Cook on Full for 15 minutes, turning the dish three times. Allow to stand for 5 minutes, then uncover and stir in the salt and soured cream. Reheat, uncovered, on Full for 2 minutes.

Herbed Beef Buffet Slice

Serves 8

900 g/2 lb/8 cups minced (ground) beef

2 large eggs, beaten

1 beef stock cube

1 small onion, finely grated

60 ml/4 tbsp plain (all-purpose) flour

45 ml/3 tbsp tomato ketchup (catsup)

10 ml/2 tsp dried mixed herbs

10 ml/2 tsp soy sauce

Mint leaves and peeled orange slices, to garnish

Thoroughly combine all the ingredients except the soy sauce. Spread into a 1¼ litre/2 pt/5 cup greased rectangular dish shaped like a loaf tin (pan). Brush the top with the soy sauce. Cover with clingfilm (plastic wrap) and slit it twice to allow steam to escape. Cook on Full for 10 minutes, then allow to stand in the microwave for 5 minutes. Cook on Defrost for a further 12 minutes, turning the dish four times. Allow to stand for 5 minutes, then uncover and carefully drain off the surplus fat and juices, which can be used for sauces and gravies. Leave until cold, then carefully transfer to a serving dish and garnish with the mint leaves and orange slices. Serve sliced.

Malaysian-style Peanut Beef with Coconut

Serves 4

2 onions, finely chopped

1 garlic clove, crushed

450 g/1 lb/4 cups extra lean minced (ground) beef

125 g/4 oz/½ cup crunchy peanut butter

45 ml/3 tbsp desiccated (shredded) coconut

2.5 ml/½ tsp hot pepper sauce

15 ml/1 tbsp soy sauce

2.5 ml/½ tsp salt

300 ml/½ pt/1¼ cups boiling water

175 g/6 oz/1½ cups rice, boiled

Oriental pickles, to garnish (optional)

Place the onions, garlic and beef into a 1.5 litre/2½ pt/6 cup casserole dish (Dutch oven). Mix together well with a fork, making sure the beef is thoroughly broken up. Cover with clingfilm (plastic wrap) and slit it twice to allow steam to escape. Cook on Full for 8 minutes, turning the dish twice. Uncover and stir in all the remaining ingredients except the rice. Cover as before and cook on Full for a further 8 minutes, turning the dish three times. Allow to stand for 3 minutes. Uncover and stir, then serve with the boiled rice and oriental pickles, if wished.

Speedy Beef and Mayonnaise Loaf

Serves 6

A super dinner party main course, more luxurious than you would expect from a dish so quick to prepare.

750 g/1½ lb/6 cups lean minced (ground) beef

15 ml/1 tbsp dried red and green (bell) pepper flakes

15 ml/1 tbsp finely chopped parsley

7.5 ml/1½ tsp onion salt

30 ml/2 tbsp plain (all-purpose) flour

60 ml/4 tbsp thick mayonnaise

7.5 ml/1½ tsp mustard powder

5 ml/1 tsp soy sauce

Thoroughly grease a deep 20 cm/8 in diameter dish. Combine the beef with all the remaining ingredients and spread smoothly into the dish. Cover with clingfilm (plastic wrap) and slit it twice to allow steam to escape. Cook on Full for 12 minutes, turning the dish four times. Allow to stand for 5 minutes, then lift the loaf out of the dish with two spatulas, leaving the fat behind. Transfer to a warmed serving plate and cut into six wedges to serve.

Beef Cooked in Red Wine

Serves 4

A smart and stylish dish, especially when served with Classic Macaroni Cheese or Savoyard Potatoes and perhaps canned artichoke hearts, warmed through in a little butter.

30 ml/2 tbsp butter or margarine

2 large onions, grated

1 garlic clove, crushed

125 g/4 oz button mushrooms, thinly sliced

450 g/1 lb rump (tip) steak, cut into small cubes

15 ml/1 tbsp tomato purée (paste)

15 ml/1 tbsp chopped parsley

15 ml/1 tbsp cornflour (cornstarch)

5 ml/1 tsp strong made mustard

300 ml/½ pt/1¼ cups dry red wine

5 ml/1 tsp salt

Put the butter or margarine in a 20 cm/8 in diameter casserole dish (Dutch oven). Melt, uncovered, on Defrost for 1–1½ minutes. Stir in the onions, garlic and mushrooms. Cook, uncovered, on Full for 5 minutes. Stir in the steak, then move the mixture to the edge of the dish to form a ring, leaving a small hollow in the centre. Cover with a plate and cook on Full for 5 minutes. Meanwhile, mix together the tomato purée, parsley, cornflour and mustard. Blend smoothly with a little of the red wine, then stir in the remainder. Mix gently into the steak mixture. Cover with a plate and cook on Full for 5 minutes, stirring twice. Allow to stand for 3 minutes. Stir in the salt, then serve.

CPSIA information can be obtained
at www.ICGtesting.com
Printed in the USA
LVHW081520100222
710600LV00011B/340

9 781804 500057